the
intelligent
man's
guide to **HAIR
TRANSPLANTS**
and other
methods
of hair
replacement

the
intelligent
man's
guide to **HAIR
TRANSPLANTS**
and other
methods
of hair
replacement

Dr. Walter P. Unger
and Sidney Katz

Library of Congress Cataloging in Publication Data

Unger, Walter P.   1939–
    The intelligent man's guide to hair transplants and other methods of hair replacement.

    Includes index.
    1. Hair—Transplant.   2. Baldness.   3. Hair—Care and hygiene.   I. Katz, Sidney, M., joint author.   II. Title.   III. Title: Hair replacement.
    RD121.5.U54   1979   617'.477   79-4500
    ISBN 0-8092-7436-1

Published by Contemporary Books, Inc.
180 North Michigan Avenue, Chicago, Illinois 60601
Manufactured in the United States of America
Library of Congress Catalog Card Number: 79-4500
International Standard Book Number: 0-8092-7436-1

Published simultaneously in Canada by
Beaverbooks
953 Dillingham Road
Pickering, Ontario L1W 1Z7
Canada

Contents

2112859

Introduction

Millions of men all over the world have decided that they are unhappy with bald heads and have determined to replace their lost hair. If you are reading this book you are probably one of them. Some of you are mildly concerned, others can think of little else, but all of you share the same problem: How do you get objective information on the various forms of hair replacement that are available today?

If you go to people who sell hairpieces, they will tend to tell you all of the good things about hairpieces and few of the bad, and similarly the purveyors of hair weaving, hair implants, and various progressive-sounding "new" methods. If you go to a "clinic" that offers you any route you prefer, it will often try to persuade you to use whichever methods it is best equipped to provide or whichever alternative it feels will produce the most profit. Or you may turn to one of the miracle "cures" for baldness that pop up incessantly.

How can the average person get accurate and unbiased information, not only about the above alternatives, but also about the complex medical solutions, such as hair transplanting, flaps, and alopecia reduction? This book is intended to give you the information you need in order to make the decision that is right for you. A major portion of the book is devoted to hair transplanting, but that is because hair transplanting is by far the most complex and difficult alternative to explain. It is also the alternative that seems to be the most grossly distorted by the media and by rumor.

However, bad experiences with hair transplanting do occur. Although the results can be excellent and the procedure surprisingly comfortable, if you have chosen the wrong doctor you can find yourself with enormous problems. One of the objectives of this book is to teach you how to find the right doctor.

For some time, I debated with myself whether or not I should write this book. The book could be viewed as personal advertising, albeit indirect advertising, and I am a staunch opponent of professionals advertising themselves. However, what finally overcame my reluctance was the recent avalanche of misleading, deceptive advertising about hair restoration by clinics and some physicians. At present, I feel that the public simply doesn't have enough authoritative information conveniently available to assess the claims and counterclaims.

As my collaborator for this work, I chose Sidney Katz, a widely experienced journalist, author, and broadcaster who specializes in the field of health. His medical articles and books have earned him an enviable reputation for accurate and balanced reporting, and I hope that his contribution has helped me to give you as unbiased a book as is possible.

the
intelligent
man's
guide to HAIR
TRANSPLANTS
and other
methods
of hair
replacement

1

What You Should Know About Losing Your Hair

If you're a male in your thirties, there's about a 40-percent chance that your family or friends will have noticed that your hair is thinning. If you're in your forties, the odds go up to about 50 percent. And, with each additional year of aging, the probability of your visibly showing the signs of balding increases.

Your father and grandfather, like most people of their generations, philosophically resigned themselves to the loss of hair. After all, what could they do about it? They derived what comfort they could from repeating such homilies as "Baldness is a sign of male virility" or "You can't grow hair over a busy brain."

But a growing number of men today are unwilling to accept the idea that they must remain bald. They're aware that, thanks to advances in public health, medicine, nutrition, cosmetics, and fashion, it's now possible to feel and look youthful well into middle age and beyond. And an essential part of the youthful look is the possession of a fine head of hair.

If you're balding, your search for attractive hair can prove confusing and frustrating because of the many alternatives available.

You may be tempted by the seductive advertisements of the hair and scalp "studios" that "guarantee" to arrest falling hair and restore hair growth. These studios rely heavily on such external treatments as heat application, massage, shampoos, and various lotions. Or, if you want to act on your own, you can go out and buy the latest miracle chemical formula on sale and hope for the best.

Another possibility is to get fitted with one of several varieties of hairpieces, formerly referred to indelicately as toupees or wigs. Still another choice is hair transplantation, the main subject of this book. The list of alternatives gets longer yearly.

Which solution is best for you? How can you avoid spending valuable time and money on solutions to your hair problem that are useless and perhaps injurious? Let's begin by giving you a few basic scientific facts about the nature of hair growth and hair loss. You should then be in a position to make an intelligent evaluation of any treatment for baldness that is said to stop hair loss or cause lost hair to regrow.

The most important thing to realize is that the odds are at least 99.99 out of 100 that your baldness is due to factors over which you have no control whatsoever. Unless you're the rare exception, you're the victim of Male Pattern Alopecia, more commonly referred to as Male Pattern Baldness, or simply MPB. At some point in your life — usually in your early twenties — your front hairline recedes, and later a tiny bald spot appears on top of your head. Ominously, the spot spreads with the passage of time.

No two people with MPB will grow bald in exactly the same way or at exactly the same speed. However, extensive observation has revealed that hair loss usually occurs in certain general sequences. Dr. James B. Hamilton, a U.S. dermatologist, has described eight typical categories of baldness (Fig. 1).

If you examine categories I to III, you'll notice that here hair loss occurs particularly at the front of the head at the hairline, or the frontotemporal region. By the time a person has progressed to category III, he can't avoid recognizing that he has a balding problem.

As a person grows older, the likelihood increases that he'll also begin to lose hair at the top of his head, referred to as the "crown"

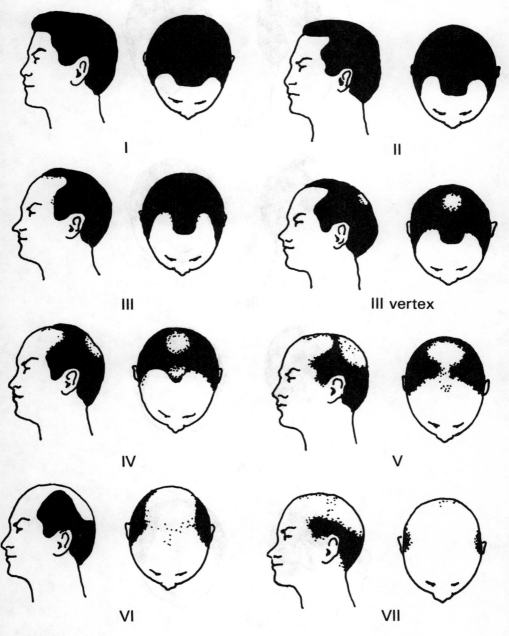

I

II

III

III vertex

IV

V

VI

VII

Fig. 1.

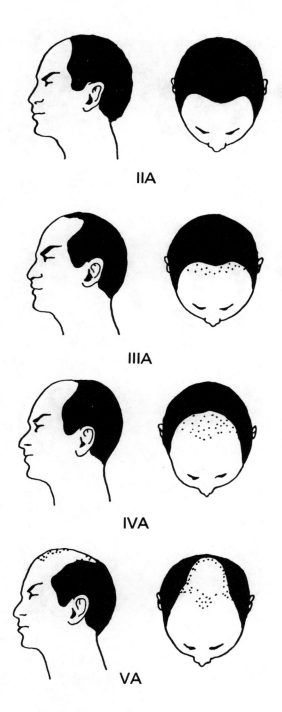

IIA

IIIA

IVA

VA

Fig. 2.

or "vertex." The stages of vertex hair loss are shown in Figure 1, categories III vertex, IV, V, VI, and VII. The extreme baldness represented in categories VI and VII — the expansive bald spot surrounded by a horseshoe-shaped fringe of hair — is found most often among men approaching sixty years of age and beyond.

If you have Male Pattern Baldness, there's a 95 percent chance that your baldness pattern conforms to one of the eight categories shown in Figure 1. The less frequent patterns of baldness — designated as "Type A Variants" — are illustrated in Figure 2.

If you want to pin responsibility for your hair loss on somebody or something, then blame your sex, your parents, or your age.

Sex.   Your sex plays a significant role, because males are the main victims of MPB.

MPB depends on the presence, in the body, of a group of male sex hormones that are referred to collectively as "androgens." Although the androgen level of bald men is no higher than that of men who are not bald, the fact remains that a certain minimum amount of androgens must be present before this type of hair loss can occur.

The average, normal man has enough androgens circulating in his body to develop MPB. Eunuchs — castrated males whose bodies no longer manufacture normal levels of androgens — have luxuriant heads of hair which they never lose. Women will seldom suffer MPB to the same degree as men, primarily because their androgen levels are usually not high enough to produce this effect. Exceptions to this general rule include: (1) Women who are on certain oral contraceptives that contain androgens. The newer "minipills" are worse in this regard than some of the older oral contraceptives. (2) Certain women in whom normal levels of circulating androgens are converted into a stronger male hormone by the individual hairs of the scalp. (This will be explained in greater detail below.) (3) Women whose production of the female hormone estrogen decreases (for example, after menopause).

Estrogen seems to counteract to a variable degree the MPB effect of androgens. Falling estrogen production "sets loose" the tendency to MPB in women who inherit the gene that causes it. Estrogen pills can in some cases prevent this hair loss, but such therapy can be associated with a large number of undesirable side effects, including an increased tendency to uterine cancer and blood clotting (which may result in strokes, phlebitis, and the like), especially in women over forty. Estrogen therapy in men can also stop hair loss if the dose is high enough, but at such levels breast enlargement, loss of libido, and hormonal problems occur.

Heredity.   The tendency to develop MPB is inherited through a gene which can come from your mother's or your father's side of the family.

The gene cannot be present in a male without producing baldness. If your father is bald, then you have a 50-percent chance of having inherited the MPB gene. However, your mother may harbor an MPB gene, but for complex reasons she may never show signs of hair thinning or baldness. All the same, she may pass the gene on to you.

If your maternal grandfather and uncles — in addition to your father — tended to lose their hair early in life, the chances are that the same fate will befall you. When I want to estimate how much hair loss a patient is likely to suffer in the years ahead, I ask him to describe the hair patterns of his male relatives on both sides of his family. Although not 100 percent foolproof, this information serves as a fairly reliable indicator.

If there's baldness among both your maternal and your paternal relatives, and you're trying to estimate how large a bald area you are going to develop (and how fast), how do you know which side of your family your MPB genes come from?

You can find clues, but again no guarantees, by examining the color and quality of your hair, rather than the quantity. If it more nearly resembles the hair of your mother's side of the family, then it's most likely that you'll follow the same balding pattern as your maternal relatives. If it's more similar to the hair of your father's side, then you're probably destined to be as bald as he is.

A word of caution: The above remarks should be regarded only as general guidelines. There are always exceptions, and in the case of any given individual, one can't predict with certainty what's going to happen to his hair. The best one can do is make an educated guess.

Something called "variable expressivity" is the reason that we can't make exact predictions about gene inheritance and hair loss. In layman's language, variable expressivity means that the MPB genes will affect some people more than others for a wide range of reasons, some known, others obscure. The MPB genes, for example, may have markedly different effects on two brothers, due to differences in their body chemistry or life-style.

To explain the vagaries of variable expressivity in another way, two brothers may come in contact with the virus that causes the common cold. However, one brother may only suffer a mild cold or "sniffles," whereas the other brother may develop a high fever and severe fatigue, and may have to take to his bed for several days. The culprit was the same cold virus in both instances, but because of individual differences in the brothers, it affected the two of them differently.

Here's another exception to the general guidelines that you should be aware of. You may be the first one in your family to develop MPB. Why this happens remains one of the many unsolved mysteries concerning hair growth and hair loss.

Age.   MPB is also linked to aging.

By the time you've reached physical maturity at 18, you have about 100,000 hairs on your head. Under normal conditions, you lose about 25 to 100 hairs per day. These are replaced by new hairs that are exactly the same in color and coarseness as the originals.

However, if you're going bald, a number of changes occur. For one, the rate of hair turnover will gradually increase, so that you will be losing and replacing hair more quickly than you once did.

Moreover, there's a change in the quality of the replacement hair. It's finer and often lighter colored, and it doesn't grow as long before falling out again.

This sequence of events takes place over and over. Men in the earliest stages of MPB notice that they no longer have to cut their hair in certain places because it doesn't grow long enough for barbering. Finally, after many such cycles, some formerly thickly growing areas on the head will be reduced to meager "peach fuzz."

Why does baldness strike one area of the head and not others?

It is likely that the cause of hair loss lies with the way each hair metabolizes or uses testosterone, the most important androgen manufactured by the body. Testosterone is in part converted by the hair into dihydrotestosterone (DHT), an even more powerful androgen. Different hairs produce differing amounts of DHT at various times. Studies in macaque monkeys have shown that the production of DHT by the individual hairs increases in balding areas at the times when hair loss is taking place and that its production falls during periods when hair loss reverts to more normal rates. At exactly the same time that DHT levels rise in the balding areas, however, they remain low in nonbalding portions of the scalp. To complicate matters further, some hairs within a balding area may not increase their production of DHT and thus are not lost. This may explain why a few hairs may remain in an otherwise bald area — their DHT production did not "follow the crowd." Women with normal estrogen and androgen levels who develop MPB probably produce more DHT in the thinning areas despite their normal blood hormone levels. Although we know about these biochemical changes, we still don't know why they happen and why some hairs will produce more DHT while hairs a few millimeters away will not.

MPB is certainly not due to a noticeable decrease in the blood supply which nourishes the scalp. If an insufficient supply of blood in certain areas resulted in hair loss, what would enable transplanted hair to flourish in these formerly bare zones?

The "decreased blood supply" explanation of baldness is now rejected by all authorities in the field. Indeed, one study suggests just the opposite — that you can slow down or stop MPB by decreasing the blood supply.

As explained earlier, testosterone is converted to DHT, which appears to be the triggering agent for hair loss. But this conversion *requires* the presence of oxygen. Theoretically, therefore, decreasing the circulation to the balding area (that is, cutting down the oxygen supply) should slow down DHT production, and therefore the balding process. Support for this theory was provided in 1972, and again in 1975, by Dr. Raymond Maréchal of Brussels, Belgium.

Working with 303 balding patients, the Belgian researcher tied off some of the main blood vessels to their scalps. This effectively cut down the scalp's blood supply, thereby reducing its supply of oxygen. Maréchal reported that an impressive 51 percent of the patients stopped losing their hair, while hair loss was slowed in an additional 21 percent.

If Maréchal's experiments were so successful, why isn't everyone tying off blood vessels as a "cure" for baldness? Because all authorities are agreed that the benefits would only be temporary. Within twelve months, the body would develop compensatory "collateral" blood vessels which would restore the blood supply to its former level. Nobody has ever shown otherwise.

Most men begin to worry about baldness when they notice several hairs sticking to the basin after a shampoo. For this reason, I want to say a few things about washing your hair and the importance — or lack of importance — of "basin hair."

Many dermatologists, including myself, believe that hair should be washed often enough to keep the scalp comfortable and free of scaling and excess oiliness. If washing it every day is necessary to achieve this effect (as may be true for persons who work on a construction site or in a big, air-polluted city), we encourage patients to do so, but we caution them to use one of the milder shampoos on the market to avoid drying out the hair shafts excessively. Whether frequent washing of an oily, dirty, or uncomfortable scalp can decrease the "natural" rate of hair loss — as is sometimes claimed — remains to be proven, though many of us feel that this may be the case. On the other hand, you can be certain that you will not go bald faster because of too frequent washing. That's an old wives' tale you should try to forget.

Some men go into a panic after noticing more than a few hairs in the basin after they've had a shampoo. They gloomily visualize themselves as going completely bald in a matter of months, if not weeks. Let me offer some words of comfort. Balding is seldom a rapid-fire process. For a time, your hair thins out. Then you hit a plateau — a time when no further thinning occurs — and this is followed by another episode of hair thinning. The "waves" of hair loss last anywhere from a few weeks to several years; the duration of the plateaus can also vary greatly. But if you're destined to go bald, it will usually happen gradually.

It's not always simple to assess the significance of basin hair.

Even if there's a residue of hundreds of hairs in the basin, you can't be sure that these hairs represent a permanent loss. You may be going through a period of acceleration of "natural turnover"; that is, the basin hairs will be replaced by an equal number of hairs of the same quality. Common causes for such accelerated hair turnover are chronic mental stress; any disease that is associated with high fever or that runs a long, chronic course of relative debilitation; postpregnancy; oral contraceptives; and certain drugs that are used mainly for the treatment of cancer. Accelerated turnover can also be caused by amphetamines, antithyroid drugs, and some anticoagulants (blood thinners). Hair loss usually occurs three to six weeks after the causal phenomenon, and it can last anywhere from a few weeks to many months—especially if the "cause" is ongoing (for example, chronic mental stress). Basin hairs are only an indication of true balding if the hairs that sprout in to replace them are lighter and finer and grow for a shorter period of time until they reach their maximum length.

Simply examining the basin hairs won't give you a clue about the all-important replacement hairs. That's why I advise my patients to keep looking in the mirror rather than in the washbasin. If they're headed for MPB, they'll notice that their hair is growing sparser and sparser. If they're simply experiencing a period of accelerated natural turnover, their hair will thin out initially (usually for a period of three to twelve months at most) but will ultimately return to the same thickness.

The Role of Diet

In the past few years, the theory of a nutritional cause for baldness has gained considerable popularity. It's claimed that balding people can slow down, stop, and even reverse their hair loss by supplementing their diet with certain vitamins, minerals, and proteins.

Proponents of this theory claim that although we are surrounded by an abundance of nutritious foods, a high proportion of the population is malnourished. Some of us are ignorant of sound eating habits. Others are too busy to eat properly. And at any given time numerous men and women are on self-prescribed and nutritionally disastrous weight-reducing diets.

In fact, it is possible that many of us who think we are eating well are missing out on certain vitamins and minerals because they're found chiefly in foods that are uncommon or unappetizing. Members of the vitamin B family spring to mind. Unless you're in the habit of eating eggs or liver *every* day or you enjoy brewer's yeast, rice polish, or a few other unfamiliar food items, there's a fair chance that on many days you're getting less than the physician-recommended daily quantity of vitamins B_6 and B_{12}.

Many nutritionists are sharply critical of the physician-recommended levels of vitamins, minerals, and proteins. They point out that although the prescribed doses may prevent illness, they're not large enough to promote optimum health. A higher daily intake of various nutrients, they claim, would yield many health benefits, including the stoppage—or the reversal—of hair loss. Vitamin E, biotin, and inositol (a deficiency of any of these may cause hair loss in rats) as well as vitamin A, iron, zinc, niacin, iodine, folic acid, vitamin B_{12}, vitamin B_3, and vitamin B_5 have been frequently marketed as "hair restorers."

These claims have yet to be proven to the satisfaction of the medical profession by double-blind, controlled scientific studies in humans.

Despite the above, however, this much must be recognized:

1. While "nutritionist" theories have not been proven by scientific studies in humans, neither have they been disproven by such studies; that is, the theories just could be right.

2. Many people do *not* eat properly; that is, they do not consume even the physician-recommended doses of all the vitamins, minerals, and proteins necessary for good health.

3. Vitamin, mineral, and protein supplements to your diet may not be helpful in stopping MPB, but if they are prescribed by a physician they will at least be safe and they will improve your general health if your diet was previously inadequate.

In summary, there is nothing to lose by taking doctor-prescribed vitamin-mineral pills and drinking three glasses of milk per day (for "essential" protein), but don't count on its helping to stop or cure MPB. No scientific study to date has supported this claim.

2

Hair Replacement: The Choices Open to You

Like many modern men, you have decided that you don't want to go around with a severely receded hairline or a noticeable bald spot. Your reasons may be economic, social, or psychological. But whatever they are, your next step is to select a method of hair replacement that best suits your particular needs. For your convenience, here's a condensed account of the main methods of hair replacement available to you.

The Hair and Scalp Studios

Every city has one or more thriving "hair studios," proof that a surprisingly large number of bald men believe that these studios hold some miraculous cure for Male Pattern Baldness. It's a misplaced faith. If you're balding or bald, there's nothing a hair studio can do for you that your family doctor or dermatologist can't do better and less expensively. Studio treatment programs — which can cost as much as $800 a year—tend to be prolonged and expensive, and they usually end in failure.

The studio "therapist"—a person without training at a recognized medical school—makes frequent use of scalp shampooing. He creates the impression that frequent cleansing of the hair and scalp will somehow put an end to hair loss and stimulate the growth of new hair. That's an unrealistic expectation. As was mentioned in the previous chapter, it's wise to keep your scalp clean and comfortable, but shampooing—even ten times a day—won't sprout a crop of bushy hair on your head. In the long run, the amount of hair you have will be determined by your sex, your age, and your genes, not by the cleanliness of your head.

Another favorite studio treatment is the application of heat and massage to the scalp. Balding, explains the therapist, is caused by "poor circulation" and the "decreased blood supply" conducted through the blood vessels in the scalp, resulting in starvation of the hair. Heat and massage presumably dilate the blood vessels and thus stimulate a greater blood supply. This, in turn, nourishes the hair and removes "toxins" or "poisons."

Unfortunately, as has already been pointed out, scientific evidence is totally lacking to support this theory of Male Pattern Baldness—and that's the kind most men have.

You may have asked yourself, "If this is true, how do the hair studios manage to survive and even prosper?" There are several explanations.

First, a small proportion of the men who come to studios for help—a very small proportion—will have suffered hair loss because of specific medical disorders. Some of these conditions eventually improve on their own, but the studios will claim credit for the improvement. Still other conditions will respond only to medication.

But keep in mind that a competent physician is better qualified than the studios to attend to all of the diseases that cause hair loss. He has the necessary skill to diagnose your condition. Furthermore, unlike the studio operator, he is legally empowered to write prescriptions for certain effective drugs when they're required.

It's also true that studios enhance their reputations by exploiting, to their advantage, the sporadic progress of Male Pattern Baldness.

As I've mentioned before, hair loss comes in waves. You go through a period of hair loss, and then for several weeks, months, or years no further thinning takes place. If a period of stabilization happens to coincide with the time you're a studio client, the operator will claim credit for the "progress" you have made.

Once you stop losing your hair, you may decide (against the studio operator's advice) to discontinue treatment. When the next wave of hair loss occurs, you may panic and rush back to the studio. There you may very well be told that your hair loss recurred because you stopped treatment. What the average layman doesn't know is that both the "plateau" and the next wave of hair loss would have occurred with or without the costly ministrations of the hair studio.

It's not uncommon for dermatologists to meet bald men who have wasted hundreds and even thousands of dollars on studio treatment. Many of these were inclined to break off treatment after a dozen or so sessions failed to show appreciable results. The studio operator persuaded them to continue, arguing, "After all, it's taken you several years to lose your hair. Isn't it unreasonable to expect to get it back in only a few months?"

To be totally fair, not all "trichologists" are frauds—just those who claim or strongly imply that they can stop or reverse MPB. A small number limit themselves to helping you select a regimen of hair and scalp care appropriate for you and your lifestyle. (They will review your general health, nutrition, environmental expo- sure—job, hobbies, sports, etc.—and how you treat your hair before suggesting a new approach and different products.) A good dermatologist or a hairdresser can do the same thing but rather sadly few seem interested enough to do it. Again some trichologists are better than others and what they can do for you will therefore vary greatly; they can be next to useless or remarkably successful in helping you improve damaged hair or a troublesome scalp. Your best route to one of these individuals (if there is a reliable one near you) is via a referral from a dermatologist, your doctor, hairdresser, or a satisfied client, in that order of preference.

The "Miracle Formulas"

If you have a hair loss problem, from time to time you've probably grown curious about—or actually tried—a highly touted new compound that is "guaranteed" to grow hair. These panaceas appear with unerring regularity in every major city throughout the world. They arouse false hopes among the bald, and then, after a period of discussion and controversy, they vanish, never to be heard from again. Beware of photographic tricks (see Figs. 12A-B and 13A-B).

Let me give you some down-to-earth advice about these highly publicized "cures" for baldness.

Sit back and wait. Don't rush out and try them. After all, you've been living with some degree of baldness for several years, so why the hurry now? The odds are less than one in a million that the new treatment will be of value.

I urge caution because the promoters of the new elixirs are usually individuals without a scientific or medical background. They fail to supply satisfactory evidence that their product is effective, or for that matter, that it's even safe. The formula is usually kept a deep, dark secret. What guarantees does the consumer have, for example, that the formula does not contain ingredients which can do injury to the body by absorption through the skin?

I should mention that in the past few years there have been several products on the market, *some promoted by physicians,* that have produced *some* hair growth. Usually, these have been used in conjunction with other treatments, such as massage and heat.

I would like to note two features of the hair produced by the new chemicals cum heat treatment. First, the hair growth is only temporary. Second, it's often not regular, healthy hair, but a short, downy fuzz known medically as "vellus" hair.

Some of the new products perform even better and produce "terminal" hair, which is coarser, thicker, and longer than vellus hair—that is, normal adult hair. Physicians regard the development of these preparations to be scientifically significant, but to date the preparations have never produced enough terminal hair to provide a cosmetically satisfactory result. After three to twelve months of conscientiously applying the baldness "cure" to his scalp, the patient will have some terminal hair on his head but will still look bald (Figs. 3A and 3B). Continuing the treatment for an additional year or two with any of the products I'm aware of brings no further improvement. (Don't let them persuade you to continue

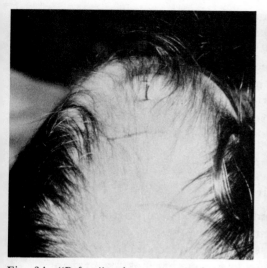

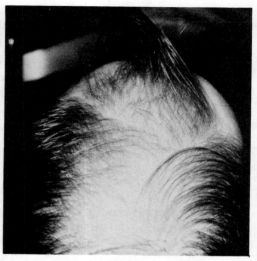

Fig. 3A. "Before" using a new "miracle formula" for growing hair. This patient applied the substance twice a day, following each application by wrapping his head in a hot towel for fifteen to twenty minures. A shampoo, a conditioner, and vitamins were also part of the program. The suture near the front of the patient's scalp was the site of a skin biopsy which was part of a study.

Fig. 3B. Six months later there was a marked increase in the amount of coarse "adult" hair present. This was not just "fuzz"; a second biopsy confirmed these positive results. If progress had continued at this rate for another six to twelve months, the patient would have had a full head of hair. Unfortunately, despite enthusiastic follow-up treatment, no further growth occurred. After twelve months the patient was fed up with the routine and the lack of further progress and gave up the program. All of the "new" hair promptly fell out. There are numerous products that have shown an *initial* "miracle" response which later peters out.

expensive treatments with the argument that "Rome wasn't built in a day.") Even the limited hair growth that is achieved by the new products will last only as long as you continue treatment. I urge you not to spend money on a preparation until there's valid evidence that it can grow a *presentable* head of hair. When such a product is discovered, your physician will recommend it without delay.

Meanwhile, you might be heartened to learn that reputable investigators are trying a variety of hormone preparations aimed at stopping MPB or regrowing lost hair. In Chapter 1, you will recall,

I mentioned that estrogens can suppress the androgens that play such an important role in MPB. However, estrogens taken orally at levels sufficient to affect MPB produce unwanted side effects. Estrogens applied directly to the scalp produce fewer side effects and may be effective in some women — in men they still result in too many significant problems. Various other chemicals that suppress or compete with androgen activity are also being tried. Thus far, unfortunately, they too are associated with unacceptable side effects, but research is continuing.

Hairpieces

Many victims of MPB will find a hairpiece a satisfactory answer to their problem. If you want guidance on where to obtain a hairpiece, consult your dermatologist or your hairdresser. Better still, if you know someone who's wearing a hairpiece that looks natural and pleasing, ask him where he got it.

In general, the modern hairpiece has succeeded the wig. The principal virtue of the wig is that it fits on the head like a helmet and is therefore more difficult to dislodge than the hairpiece. The wig can also effectively cover total baldness. But it has drawbacks. A wig is heavier and warmer than a hairpiece, and it often lacks naturalness. A man of fifty-five, for example, sporting the luxuriant hair of a youth of twenty-five is apt to be conspicuous.

Hairpieces on the market today can be of domestic or foreign manufacture, and they usually range in price from $50 to $1,500. Naturally, the larger the hairpiece, the more costly it is. Hairpieces are made of synthetic or human hair, or a combination of both. The most acceptable hairpieces on the market are composed of at least 40 percent human hair. Because human hair has a more natural appearance than synthetic hair, the higher the proportion of human hair used, the more natural looking (and expensive) the hairpiece. On the other hand, the synthetic products are more durable than the natural products and have to be replaced less frequently.

A hairpiece consists of hairs or hairlike fibers attached to a light, thin cloth or plasticized mesh which "breathes" easily through small holes. It's affixed to the head by strips of transparent tape with adhesive on both sides. Most wearers remove the hairpiece at night when they go to bed, and stick it back on again in the morning with fresh strips of tape. The adhesive is strong enough to keep the hairpiece firmly in place during routine activities.

A new type of hairpiece, especially designed for strenuous activities and swimming, has recently come on the market. It's composed entirely of sturdy synthetic hair, firmly mounted on a water-repellent silicone base. Since the hairpiece doesn't breathe, the wearer would be uncomfortably warm wearing it in a heated room. The "sports model" hairpiece is glued to the scalp with a liquid adhesive containing silicone. To remove it, you work your fingers all the way around the edge, pressing firmly, and it pops loose. Most of the people who buy one of these hairpieces also buy a more standard "breathing" model, using the sports model only when they are engaged in strenuous activity.

Because I want to avoid being guilty of overselling the hairpiece as a method of hair replacement, let me list some of its disadvantages:

1. All hairpieces are hot and uncomfortable on a torrid summer day or in a warm room. True, the newer models have "breathing holes" in their bases, which are an improvement, but some uncomfortable warmth still exists.

2. Hairpieces must be taken off periodically, and the trauma of seeing yourself bald in the mirror is ego-deflating.

3. There's always the anxiety that your hairpiece might go flying in impromptu sports, or when you're making love. (As was mentioned earlier, the rugged sports model hairpiece is not designed for everyday use.)

4. Attractive, high-quality hairpieces are costly, ranging in price from $500 to $1,500. The most expensive and natural-looking ones—those made entirely of human hair—often last a year or less. Hairpieces containing a sizable proportion of synthetic materials have to be replaced after three or four years.

There are also other expenses. You need two hairpieces—one to wear while the other is being cleaned. In addition, you may want to use an "action" hairpiece. And, of course, every few weeks there's a charge for the cleaning.

5. The front hairline of the hairpiece is straight and therefore

unnatural in appearance, because real hair doesn't grow that way. To correct this, you always have to comb the hair forward and keep the front hairs in place with a spray. (Afro hairpieces are exceptions to this generalization.)

6. If you require white hair in your hairpiece you have an additional problem. White hair yellows with time and cleaning.

Despite these disadvantages, if cost is a secondary problem, I would give a high rating to a well-made hairpiece that has 75 to 100 percent human hair, is well matched to the patient's hair color, and is mounted on a webbed base. Such a hairpiece should be cleaned regularly and be replaced every one to two years.

In my opinion, a good hairpiece is cosmetically preferable to all of the other currently available alternatives with the possible exception of a good hair transplant in properly selected patients.

In an attempt to improve on the traditional hairpiece, which is affixed to the scalp with adhesive, three other techniques of attachment have been developed that I'd like to describe: hair weaving, hair implanting, and tunnel grafting. Remember that a hairpiece is used with all three of these alternatives and that the final cosmetic result depends largely on how good the hairpiece is. (Individual hair implanting will also be included in this section because of similarities it has to ordinary hair implanting, but it does not involve the use of a hairpiece.)

Hair Weaving

Instead of being stuck to the scalp with adhesive tape, in hair weaving the hairpiece is firmly tied to an "anchoring band" of tough nonshrinkable thread which is in turn tied onto the hairs in the remaining fringe of hair (Figs. 4A–4C).

This firm anchorage banishes the fear that the hairpiece will be dislodged during such activities as tennis, swimming, showering, and sex. Moreover, affixing a hairpiece by means of hair weaving is cooler than using a conventional hairpiece because there's a space between the hairpiece and the surface of your head. Hair weaving is also cooler because the base of the hairpiece is a net with fairly wide spaces between the threads, allowing air to circulate (Fig. 4B).

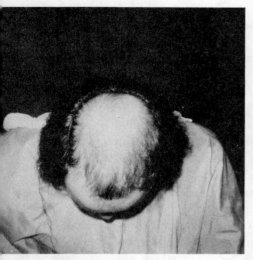

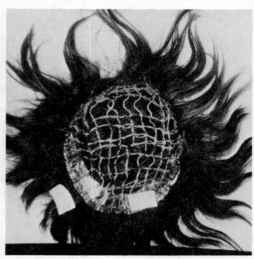

ig. 4A. An "anchoring band" of thread is
ed onto the hairs at the remaining fringe of
air.

Fig. 4B. A hairpiece with a netlike base with
large holes (for air to get in) is made to
match your own hair color and quality.

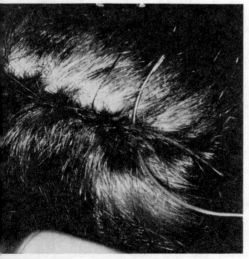

ig. 4C. The hairpiece is sewn onto the
nchoring thread with a large curved needle.

To provide you with a complete picture, here are some of the disadvantages of hair weaving:

1. It is more expensive than an ordinary hairpiece, costing between $750 and $2,000.

2. As the hair to which the anchoring thread is attached grows longer, the hairpiece grows looser on the scalp. It's therefore necessary to return to the hairpiece parlor for a "tightening," that is, to have the anchoring thread moved closer to the scalp. Since this procedure must be repeated every two to four weeks and usually costs $20 to $30, obviously hair weaving entails considerable ongoing inconvenience and expense.

3. It's very difficult for the wearer to clean properly between the hairpiece and the scalp. This results in a buildup of sebaceous secretions, skin scale, and, occasionally, annoying odors.

4. The hair on the rim of the head, to which the hairpiece is anchored, is often pulled out by traction.

5. The hairline is even less satisfactory than that of the conventional hairpiece, and the hair is not as evenly distributed, as natural looking, or as dense. This is due to the wide spaces in the net base.

Hair Implanting

To avoid the inconvenience and cost of the repeated tightenings of hair weaving, hair implanting was introduced about ten years ago.

Instead of being anchored to the fringe hairs with thread, the hairpiece is attached to Teflon-coated stainless steel sutures that are looped through the skin of the scalp and left in place there (Figs. 5A and 5B).

One variation of hair implanting does not use a hairpiece, but instead attaches wefts of hair directly to a series of concentric loops or sutures (Figs. 5C and 5D). This approach lets more air reach the scalp and is thus cooler. It also makes cleaning the scalp easier. For obvious reasons, however, it rarely produces the same density of hair as a full hairpiece attached to sutures.

In my opinion, hair implanting is to be frowned on for medical, aesthetic, practical, and financial reasons:

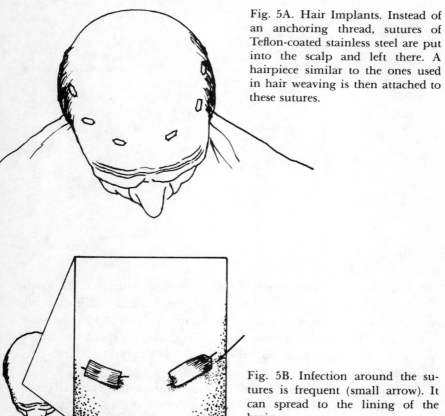

Fig. 5A. Hair Implants. Instead of an anchoring thread, sutures of Teflon-coated stainless steel are put into the scalp and left there. A hairpiece similar to the ones used in hair weaving is then attached to these sutures.

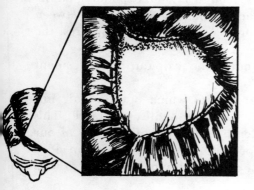

Fig. 5B. Infection around the sutures is frequent (small arrow). It can spread to the lining of the brain.

Fig. 5C. A variation of hair implanting in which more sutures are used. In this variation, wefts of hair, rather than a hairpiece, are attached to the sutures.

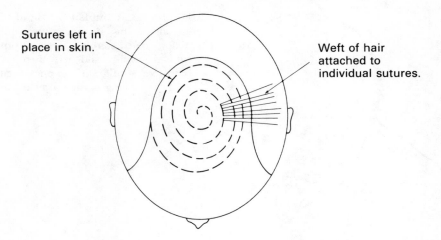

Sutures left in place in skin.

Weft of hair attached to individual sutures.

Fig. 5D.

1. Although the promoters of this procedure claim that the loops are made of "nonreacting material" and are "used in cardiovascular surgery," infections very frequently occur in the scalp at the sites where the loops are installed. Such infections can spread to other parts of the body, including the brain, causing serious and permanent damage.

2. It's very difficult to clean the scalp underneath the hairpiece adequately, resulting in physical discomfort and unpleasant odor. As was noted above, the concentric loop approach is preferable for this reason.

3. The cost is approximately $1,500 to $2,500, depending on the quality of the hair used. Considering that the difference between hair implanting and hair weaving is a matter of a few sutures, the difference in price appears to be excessive.

4. The sutures could be torn out of the scalp during an accident or a fight.

It's been my experience that studios which opt for hair implanting generally use a very cheap, poor-quality hairpiece. This enables them to make a considerably higher profit. If any of our readers unwisely elect for this procedure, the least they can do is make sure that they're getting a good-quality hairpiece to go with the sutures.

Fiber Implantation or Individual Hair Implants

Recently, several techniques have been developed in which strands of synthetic hairlike fibers are "injected" or "implanted" directly into the scalp (either singly or in clumps) to fill in the thinning or bald spots. A small knot, loop, or hook at the bottom of the strand keeps it from falling out. Thousands of synthetic fibers are implanted under local anesthesia, usually in one to three sessions, to produce "a full head of hair."

The advantages claimed for this approach are that it's a permanent solution to baldness and that it's absolutely safe. Since the synthetic material used is "nonreacting," inflammation and infection presumably "do not occur."

The facts are that it's as yet impossible to validate the claim that the implanted hair stays put indefinitely, since our experience with the technique extends only over the past few years. I recently attended a dermatology meeting during which dozens of physicians reported on numerous patients whose implanted hair started to fall out in irregular clumps after eighteen months or less. The missing hair gives the patient a moth-eaten appearance that can only be corrected by having further implants done.

But even if someone were to discover how to implant synthetic fibers into the scalp so that they remained there forever, another serious problem would arise. We have not yet developed "synthetic hair" that does not deteriorate after one to three years. Sun, wind, and chlorinated pool water; sweating, washing, combing, and blow-drying—all take their toll, and in time the synthetic hair becomes lifeless (lacking color, tone, and the like) and must be replaced.

Attempts at replacing the dull, worn fibers with fresh ones may lead to complications. If fibers are "permanently" in place, how do you get them out? What does the scalp look like when old fibers are removed? Can you insert the new fibers in the old spots? Will the scalp accept synthetic implants the second or third time around as readily as it did the first time? Ultimately, how many times will the fibers have to be replaced? Will the synthetic fibers all come out at about the same time, or will they drop out piecemeal, thus necessitating frequent trips to the clinic for repairs? If numerous "catch-up" sessions are necessary, what is the technique's ultimate total cost?

There are still some unanswered questions about the safety of individual hair implants. As we noted when we were discussing the original hair implants, a foreign material that is inserted into the scalp tends to serve as a focus around which infection can occur. The possibility of infection exists whether or not the inserted material is "nonreacting." A recent article in the *Journal of the American Medical Association* (Jan. 12, 1979) also described twenty patients all of whom lost nearly all of the implanted hair within ten weeks. Most of these individuals had problems with infection, persistent pain, facial swelling, and in many cases, subsequent scarring. While all patients will not have such unfortunate results (one clinic may be "dirtier" or less careful than another for example), the possibility of their occurrence is constant.

If an infection occurs and it is not too severe, it can be controlled by antibiotics, and if the infection is contained long enough, the body could theoretically encapsulate fibers (or sutures) in scarlike tissue and the infection could cease without the continued use of antibiotics. Despite the foregoing, one should anticipate some cases of infection when fibers are inserted directly into the scalp, and there's a chance that such infections will run out of control. There's always the possibility of severe side effects.

Time alone will provide authoritative answers to the many unanswered questions about the permanence, safety, and general desirability of hair implants. If you do investigate any of the present or future options, be sure to ask all of the questions previously noted — most important, the rate of complications, and second, the length of time that the procedure has actually been done. Remember that one can claim with certainty only that the hair will last for as long as the procedure has been applied. The rest is only speculation. In my opinion, given the present state of information, you would be wise to sit back, wait, and watch. Let somebody else experiment with his head.

Tunnel Grafts

In this approach, a rectangular strip of skin (approximately 2½ inches by ½ inch) is excised from behind one of your ears. The strip is divided in two and fashioned into two loops which are implanted in the scalp on top of the head about six to eight inches apart (one at the front of the head and one near the crown). The hairpiece is then firmly tied or clipped to these two loops, or "tunnels," of skin (Figs. 6A and 6B). Once again, the cosmetic effectiveness of the final result will depend largely on the quality of the hairpiece used.

This method is superior to hair implanting in one important respect. Since the skin loop—unlike the stainless steel loop—is derived from the patient's own body and has no open, raw surfaces when it is completed, the risk of infection is reduced to virtually nil. A disadvantage is that you may lose some scalp skin if the hairpiece gets heavily yanked.

Tunnel grafting for MPB is a disfiguring operation. You end up with two loops of skin installed on the surface of your head. For patients with very large scarred areas, however, it remains a viable alternative, as the tunnels are far less disfiguring than the scars.

Strip or Flap Grafts

In this form of hair replacement, a strip of skin ¼ to ⅓ inches wide and up to eight inches long is cut out of your permanent rim of hair. It is sewn into place in the bald area after an adequate strip of bald skin has been cut out to prepare a bed for it.

The transplanted strip may be entirely unattached to any portion of the scalp and thus be freely moved from one site to another. Or, the strip graft may remain attached at one end and simply flipped over to cover a prepared bald area. This pivoting style of graft is referred to as a "flap" graft (Fig. 7). Flap grafts can be wider than "free" strips (1½–2 inches versus ¼ to ⅓ inches).

The advantages of these procedures are:

1. Relatively large amounts of hair can be transplanted in a short period of time (one operation for a free strip, up to three operations within a period of two weeks for a flap).

2. In transplanting with strips or flaps, the results are immediately apparent. Unlike the conventional punch method of hair

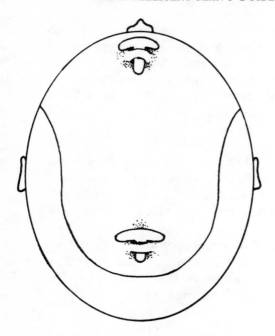

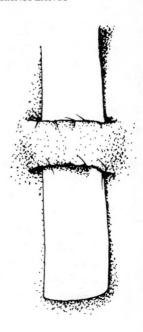

Fig. 6A. Tunnel grafting—two strips of skin taken from behind the ears are fashioned into loops and implanted at the front and back of the scalp. A hairpiece is then clipped onto these "handles" of skin.

Fig. 6B. Close-up view of th "handle" or "tunnel" immediatel after surgery. A rubber tube i running through a space lined b intact skin which is not prone to infection when it heals. The tub is left in for twenty-four hours s that clots will not bind the "han dle" down.

transplanting, strip or flap grafts are usually unaccompanied by an initial period of hair loss.

3. Hair growth is usually quite dense *with flaps*. (As is noted below, free grafts are less reliable.)

Important disadvantages of the strip and flap techniques are:

1. The hair cannot be directed in a totally natural way. If it is directed forward for example (so the hairline is not evident), it tends to lie flat down against the forehead like a bang (Fig. 8 in the color insert). Alternatively, if the strip is placed so that the hair is

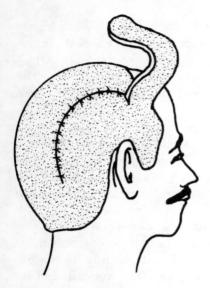

Fig. 7. A strip of skin is removed from the temple but remains attached at its front end. The "donor" site is sewn closed (above).

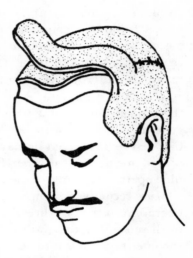

An appropriate strip of skin is cut out of the bald area and discarded (above).

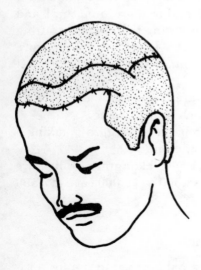

The "donor" strip is laid into place and secured with sutures (above).

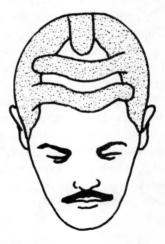

Two additional flaps (one taken from the other side of the scalp and one from the back of the head) can be done to help cover large bald areas (above).

directed toward the back of the head, the hairline is both highly visible and generally unnatural in appearance. This is the main reason I do not recommend flaps for the front of the scalp. Obviously, this problem is not nearly as serious in the mid-scalp or the crown as it is at the front hairline, and therefore flaps are more reasonable alternatives at those sites.

2. As has been noted earlier, a single flap graft usually requires three operations over a period of two weeks (the last one under a general anesthetic, with you "asleep"). When there's a large area of baldness to be covered, it may be necessary to use two or three flaps, placed one behind the other. The procedure, therefore, can require nine operations, three of them under a general anesthetic.

More recently, narrower and shorter flaps have been done in one operation instead of three. If the same area is to be covered, more of these smaller flaps will be necessary. Put differently, if you use the one-stage flaps instead of the three-stage flaps you will end up with more than one-third as many operations if you intend to cover the same-sized area.

When several flaps are used, one ends up with strips of relatively dense hair that are separated from each other by strips of bald skin. This pattern of hair growth is considerably more unnatural and therefore more limiting as regards hair styling than punch grafting is. Attempts to cut out the bare strips at a later date can improve the situation, but does not entirely eliminate the problem for most patients.

4. The scars left in the donor area are larger and more difficult to conceal than those present after punch transplanting.

5. Free strips are notoriously unreliable as regards "taking." Partial or total loss of strips is not uncommon.

6. Each strip usually costs about $1,500. Flap grafts, which are far more complicated, generally cost $2,500 to $5,000 each ($7,500 to $15,000 for three).

Excision

Sometimes the easiest way to treat a bald area is to simply cut it out. Patients who have a bald spot in the middle of an otherwise fairly heavy growth of hair can often be helped in this way (Figs. 9A

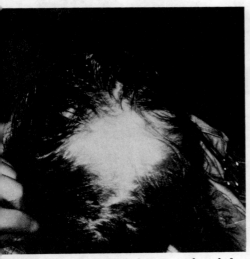

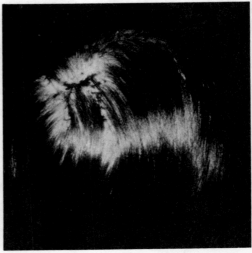

Fig. 9A. This young lady was referred for punch transplanting of a large scar on her crown. It had been caused by a burn in infancy.

Fig. 9B. Instead of punch transplanting, which would have required four operations, the bald area was cut out, producing this result with a single operation. The photo was taken one week after surgery. The remaining bald area was so small that it was easy to conceal with surrounding hair and further treatment was unnecessary.

and 9B). Such patients generally have the bald spot because of a previous infection, a disease, a burn, or other injury.

If the hairless area is small it is just cut out, and the edges of the gap are sewn together. With larger bald areas, excision must be accompanied by special plastic surgical grafting techniques that can require more than one operation.

Depending on how complicated the procedure is — and sometimes it can be very complicated — excision and grafting can cost anywhere from $200 to $2,500.

Punch Transplanting

Punch transplanting is a hair replacement technique which does not involve the use of hairpieces, loops, or any other devices. It makes use of the patient's own hair. The surgeon punches out

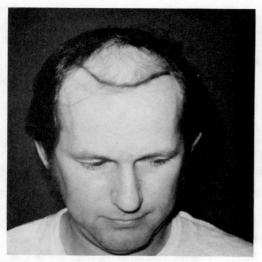

Fig. 10A. Before transplanting.

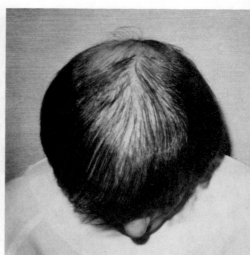

Fig. 10B. Mid-course in transplanting. Note that tufts of hair are more densely distributed in the front part, where more sessions have been done at this point. Additional transplanting was done throughout the front two-thirds of this man's scalp. (The "crown," or vertex, was not transplanted.)

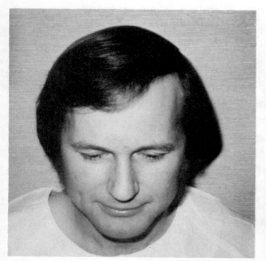

Fig. 10C. Front view fourteen months after starting transplanting.

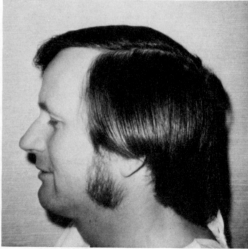

Fig. 10D. Side view after fourteen months. This patient illustrates the cosmetic benefits of punch transplanting even when it is limited to just a portion of the bald area.

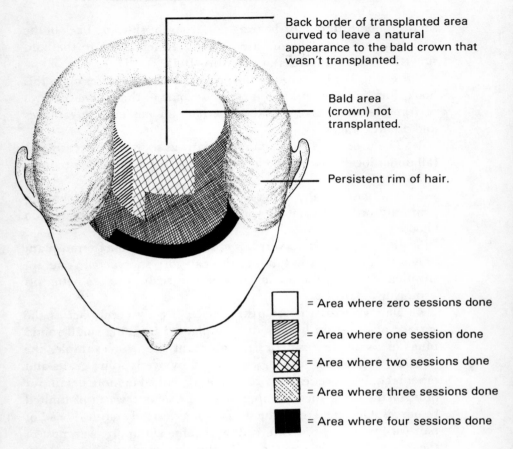

Back border of transplanted area curved to leave a natural appearance to the bald crown that wasn't transplanted.

Bald area (crown) not transplanted.

Persistent rim of hair.

☐ = Area where zero sessions done

▨ = Area where one session done

▩ = Area where two sessions done

▨ = Area where three sessions done

■ = Area where four sessions done

Fig. 10E. This patient was thirty-six at the time of his last transplant operation. We left a potential 150 to 250 grafts all around the upper few inches of his persisting rim of hair (a) because some of these areas might eventually lose their hair as he got older, i.e., they might not be permanent in their original site and therefore wouldn't be permanent wherever we had moved them to and (b) because we wanted to leave reserves of donor grafts if his baldness did extend as he got older and he needed more grafts to fill in the new bald area. (An alternate method of dealing with any new bald areas would be cutting them out—"alopecia reduction"—this is described in greater detail later in the book.)

Obviously, the younger the patient, the greater the need to leave "margins of safety" in regard to possible nonpermanence of some rim hair, and reserves for future loss.

small, round tufts of hair-bearing skin from the side and back of the patient's head (the "donor" areas) and transfers them to the bald sites (the "recipient" areas). (Figs. 10A–10E).

Since a detailed account of this technique appears later on in this book, for the moment I will merely list some of the salient features of transplanting. Like all other methods, it has both advantages and disadvantages.

1. The procedure can require as many as six to eight treatments (all under local anesthesia), spread out over a period of 9½ months or more.

2. The cost usually ranges from $750 to $10,000, depending primarily on the extent of your baldness and on the doctor you choose.

3. If your bald area is very large, it may be possible to transplant only a part of it. If you fall into this category and you can't accept the idea of a bald spot on any area of your scalp, you are better off acquiring a hairpiece.

4. Hair growth is never distributed perfectly evenly across the surface of the scalp because it is implanted by using small round plugs of tissue. In cosmetically important sites, for example, the hairline, "clumping" can be eliminated by overlapping grafts and other technical niceties. But, as will be explained in more detail, for most of the scalp such an approach represents a waste of limited resources. One can create the illusion of a perfectly natural head of hair with relatively little effort despite some clumping over most of the scalp, but it is never exactly the way you once were (Figs. 23A–23G and 24A–24D).

5. As with other cosmetic procedures, you can only obtain good results if your surgeon combines technical expertise with artistic skill. Finding such a physician can be extremely difficult for the average layman. For this reason, the entire next chapter has been devoted to that problem.

In my opinion, despite the difficulties and the disadvantages of punch transplanting, it is the treatment of choice for thousands of men with Male Pattern Baldness. After reading Chapter 4 in this book ("Are You a Good Candidate for Transplanting?"), you will be in a better position to judge whether or not you belong in this group.

One advantage of hair transplanting is that transplanted hair won't fall out or fall off no matter what kind of activity you engage in. Another is that in the hands of a competent surgeon you can depend on ending up with a very natural-looking head of hair, including a hairline that won't attract attention. Furthermore, once you've received a transplant, no further upkeep is required and no further expenses are incurred.

An estimated one million patients have received transplants since it was introduced over twenty years ago. Experience has shown that hair transplanting is a safe and — believe it or not — relatively painless procedure.

Alopecia Reduction, or Hair-Lifting

Just as excision can be used to eliminate or reduce the size of a bald scar, it can also be used to reduce an area of MPB. "Alopecia reduction," as this procedure is termed, has therefore recently become an integral part of the overall punch transplanting procedure for some patients. Alopecia reduction is generally carried out during one of the intervals between punch transplanting sessions, but it can be done before punch transplanting is started.

Essentially, a strip of skin is cut out of the bald area and the edges of the gap are then sewn together. How much can be removed depends on how "loose" the scalp is prior to the operation. The looser the better. On average, forty-five square centimeters are excised, for example, a strip just over two centimeters wide and twenty centimeters long, but some patients can have up to sixty square centimeters excised (Figs. 11A and 11B).

It takes approximately nine punch grafts to transplant one square centimeter of skin solidly. (The recipient holes are usually each 3.0 to 3.5 millimeters). The removal of forty-five square centimeters therefore produces a cosmetic improvement equivalent to that of 405 grafts. In addition, the effect is immediate. In practice, the area cut out is usually one that would not have been filled solidly with plugs (see schematic drawings accompanying photos), but the "savings" would still be approximately 200 or 300 grafts.

What does one do with these saved grafts? They can be held "in reserve" for use in bald spots that may develop later. They can be

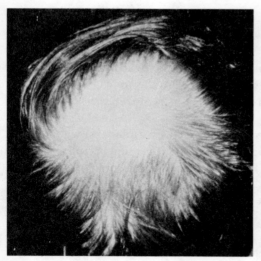 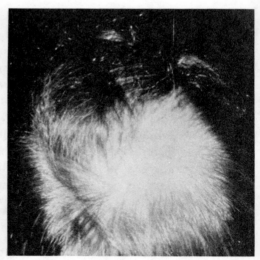

Fig. 11A. Before alopecia reduction. The front three-fourths of this patient's scalp had been transplanted (the same patient is shown in Figure 24), but the crown remained to be done. Unfortunately, there were not enough grafts left in the donor area to satisfactorily transplant such a large site.

Fig. 11B. A T-shaped area of skin was removed, and the original bald area was reduced by approximately 50 percent. There were enough remaining donor grafts to transplant this reduced area.

used to fill more densely any area being transplanted—as was mentioned earlier, most people don't have enough donor grafts available to solidly fill their entire bald area. They can be used to increase the proportion of the original bald area that can be transplanted with the number of grafts you originally thought you'd use.

Alopecia reduction can convert a patient with a very large bald area from an "unacceptable" to an "acceptable" candidate for punch transplanting. In addition, it is extremely useful in treating patients who, for a variety of reasons, have had poor transplanting results. Areas that grew very little hair can be removed. Any good grafts within the excised piece can be used to thicken the remaining transplanted areas.

The disadvantages of alopecia reduction include the following:

1. Although it can reduce the area of MPB it can rarely if ever eliminate MPB entirely.

2. Your scalp may feel somewhat tight for one to six weeks. Within six months to a year, however, it will probably have loosened up enough to allow for a second reduction if you want it.

3. The top of your head may be numb for three to twelve months.

Alopecia reduction will *not* change the shape of your head, face, or eyes. Nor will it result in a noticeable lifting of your ears.

Alopecia reduction costs between $1,000 and $1,500 at most centers. In view of the fact that the saved grafts would have cost considerably more, it represents good value to anyone who is a good candidate for it and is having punch transplanting done.

Summary. There are advantages and disadvantages to all methods of hair replacement. Although the majority of this book deals with punch hair transplanting, I do not recommend it for everyone. Having read this brief account of the alternatives, you must decide for yourself which method suits you best.

3

How to Find a Competent Hair Transplant Surgeon

You have carefully reviewed all the alternatives open to you. If you finally decide that hair transplant surgery is the best solution to your problem, your next step is to find a physician who possesses both the surgical skill and the artistic talent that are required to produce a natural and attractive result.

What kind of medical specialist should you be looking for? How do you go about finding him or her? And how can you be certain that your choice is a wise one?

The punch hair transplanting procedure was first described by a Japanese dermatologist, Dr. Shoji Okuda (in 1939), and in 1959 it was incorporated into the treatment of MPB by an American dermatologist, Dr. Norman Orentreich. For many years the procedure was carried out primarily by dermatologists.

At present, most hair transplanting is being performed by two kinds of medical specialists: dermatologists and plastic surgeons. Dermatologists are experts in disorders of the skin and hair; plastic surgeons are highly skilled in repairing and reconstructing various parts of the human body. In addition to these two groups, however, large numbers of various types of specialists (for example, general surgeons; ear, nose, and throat surgeons; and head and neck surgeons) and even family practitioners have started to transplant hair.

It is relatively unimportant whether the surgeon you choose is a dermatologist, a plastic surgeon, an ear, nose, and throat specialist, or for that matter not a specialist at all. What is important is that he has had adequate training and experience in punch transplanting. Any physician who meets the requirements outlined in this chapter should be acceptable to you.

The best place to begin your search for the person who's going to recreate your hair pattern is in the office of your family doctor. Ask him whether he knows of a competent physician who specializes in hair transplantation. He may not. He may even think that cosmetic surgery of any type borders on the disgraceful—and he may let you know it. On the other hand, he is in the best position to find several transplant specialists for you to consult with. Try to persuade him to get those names for you—whether or not he likes cosmetic surgery.

For reasons of convenience and economics it's wisest to be treated by a doctor who lives in your community. However, if you live in a small center, the chances are that you'll have to travel elsewhere to have your transplant done.

Another approach is to phone, write, or visit the offices of your local, state, or provincial medical association, and to ask for a list of the members who perform this operation. Although medical associations generally decline to endorse an individual doctor, most have no objection to providing you with a panel of names to choose one from.

For people who live in the United States or Canada, the American Society for Dermatologic Surgery (ASDS) is yet another source of names of prospective transplant specialists. The members of this society are dermatologists, plastic surgeons, and other physicians who, as the society's name implies, have a specific interest in skin surgery—including hair transplanting. Inquiries can be sent to the current secretary of the society, Dr. Daniel Gormley, 210 South Grand Avenue, Glendora, California 91740. Some non-North

American surgeons are also members of the ASDS, and it might be worthwhile to contact the society, regardless of where you live.

Select a doctor, and phone for an appointment to discuss the possibility of a hair transplant. The interview serves a double purpose. You have the opportunity to judge the suitability of the doctor; the doctor, in turn, can decide whether or not you're a suitable candidate for a hair transplant.

During the interview, don't have any compunctions about asking questions about the operation or about the doctor and his qualifications. After all, it's your health, your head, and your appearance that are at stake, and what can be of greater importance to you? A doctor of good reputation who has confidence in his professional ability will be only too happy to discuss his work and his qualifications.

Admittedly, it's generally difficult for a layman such as yourself to assess the competence and suitability of a surgeon. Nor is the task made any easier by physicians who are annoyed by patients who are obviously trying to assess their medical capabilities. A reasonable amount of tact and courtesy is therefore indicated.

In the case of all cosmetic surgery, especially with hair transplants, you can judge how good a surgeon is by carefully examining photos of his results. In some cosmetic procedures, the physician will object to showing photos on the ground that it would reveal the identity of his patients. However, the faces of hair transplant patients can be entirely blacked out.

The physician may also point out that it is difficult to find a photograph of a patient whose hair and hair problem were exactly the same as yours, so that none of his photos provide an accurate representation of the result you might expect. That's a valid objection. However, if you are shown enough "before" and "after" photos, you should get some idea of what your prospects are, even though an exact replica of your situation may not be available. Except for seeing a patient in person, I know of no better way to judge a doctor's handiwork than by comparing colored distant and close-up pictures of patients before and after his operations.

But photos may mislead you if you don't know what you're looking at.

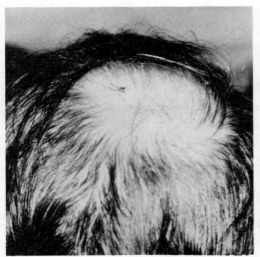

Fig. 12A. Before.

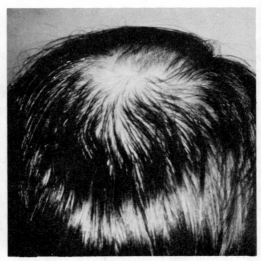

Fig. 12B. This is the patient shown in Figure 12A, but the photo has been taken with less light and the head is tilted ten to fifteen degrees farther forward. As a result the bald spot looks hairier and much smaller.

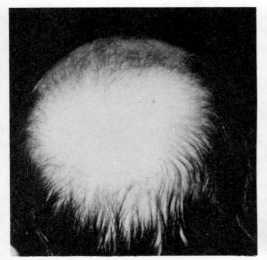

Fig. 13A. Before.

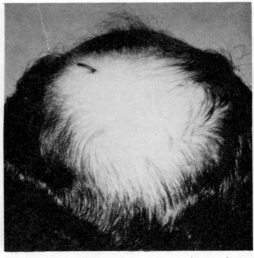

Fig. 13B. The same patient, but photographed with less light and with the head tipped ten to fifteen degrees farther forward.

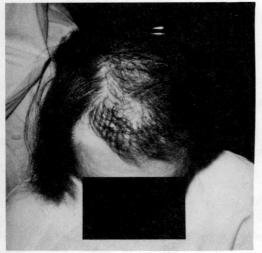

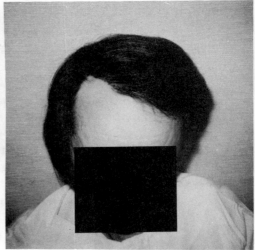

Fig. 14A. Patient with two hair transplanting sessions growing at the front of the thinning area. Note the long hair to his right side. By parting his hair one to two inches lower than the thin area, this patient is able to comb the long hair over it, producing a thicker appearance. This styling also helps camouflage the transplanted area during the healing stages after each operation.

Fig. 14B. The same patient as shown in Figure 14A, with his long hair combed in place.

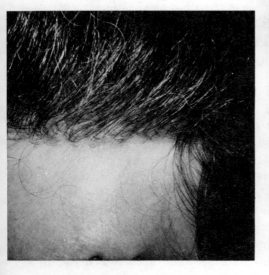

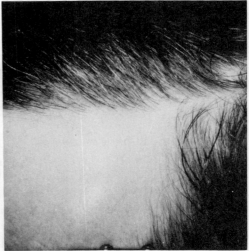

Fig. 15A. Close-up of a transplanted hairline with the hair falling forward naturally.

Fig. 15B. The same hairline with the hair combed up to fully expose the hairline. Photographs such as these are not significantly effected by changes in lighting, angle, or grooming techniques, and are therefore your best way of estimating how good the doctor's work can be.

A good surgeon may be a poor photographer, and the results shown in the "after" photos may quite accidentally appear to be better than they actually are. As an example, you may be shown an "after" picture of the crown in which the head is tilted forward at a sharper angle than in the "before" picture (Figs. 12A and 12B). Even a slight amount of tilting can create the illusion of a much smaller bald spot. Again, darker lighting in the "after" picture can create the impression that the hair is thicker than it really is (Figs. 13A and 13B).

You should also be on the lookout for photos in which the bald or thin spots have been camouflaged by special efforts in combing or brushing the hair. Parting the hair an inch or two lower, for example, can instantly "grow" hair (Figs. 14A and 14B). Many patients who are asked to come in for "after" photos are so proud of their new hair that they go to great lengths to wash, blow-dry, and style it in order to give the surgeon as much satisfaction as he has given them. Although the photos are not intentionally deceptive, the patients may look better in them than they usually look. But good hair styling is an adjunct to transplanting. It is quite legitimate to show "after" photos that incorporate it — as long as you are aware of what styling techniques are being used in each case.

Give your most careful attention to the photographs of the hairline. (See Figs. 15A and B, 17D, and 21C. In the color insert, see Figs. 18A and 18B, 19, and 20.) The crucial test of both the skill and the artistry of the physician is his ability to create a hairline that is natural looking. A close-up of the hairline, with the hair combed up to expose it fully, will tell you beyond a doubt how good the doctor really is. In general I would advise you to never proceed with any physician who cannot provide adequate hairline photos. The exception to this rule would be a well-trained doctor who has just begun private practice and who therefore would not have an extensive collection of photos, even though he might be able to produce good results. You should also remember that how good the hair transplanting (and hairline) is, will not only depend on how skilled the doctor is but also will vary with how dense the hair in the donor area is, skin coloring, hair coloring, and how well the patient heals. This is explained more fully later. Photographs showing you end results of transplanting will only be able to be used by you as a form of assurance that given the right combination of these factors, your doctor is capable of producing good results. The more good hairline photos he can show you, with differing types of hair texture and color, etc., the more confident you can be of his ability.

In addition to examining "before" and "after" photographs, you should spend some time during the interview trying to obtain answers to the following four questions:

1. *Does the doctor possess good medical credentials?* In addition to having graduated from a good medical school, your doctor should ideally possess a specialist's certificate in dermatology, plastic surgery, or some related specialty. This assures you that he's had at least three years of intensive medical training, under supervision, following his graduation from medical school. If he holds — or has held — a post on the staff of an accredited hospital, that's an additional indication of professional merit.

2. *Does the doctor enjoy a good medical reputation?* You can begin by inquiring about him from other physicians or from patients he's treated, if you're fortunate enough to know of any.

You should be wary of a physician who has "gone commercial" and blatantly advertises his services with ads in newspapers and magazines. In some countries, even billboard advertising by doctors has become common!

The medical profession has always frowned on advertising — and for good reasons. Much as the public would prefer otherwise, medical treatment is generally too complex for laymen to be able to judge it competently. Instead, for example, the profession has always left it to the family practitioner to judge for his patients which specialists are best and to refer accordingly. The patient who goes to someone who has advertised hair transplanting or any other medical service may find that he has gone to the doctor with the largest advertising budget rather than the best doctor.

Recently the courts in many localities have ruled that advertising by professionals is legal and further, that it is illegal for professional societies to penalize their members for advertising. You must therefore expect to see more and more advertising by "hair transplanting specialists," either directly or via companies that will provide whatever method of hair replacement you may want, be it hairpieces, hair weaves, implants, transplants, and so on. It would be very wise of you to remember that a top-rated surgeon has no need to hawk his skills and that he would be unlikely to affiliate himself with organizations or services that use high-pressure methods of promoting him. If a doctor is good, he's kept busy by patients who come to him directly because of word-of-mouth advertising or by patients whom other physicians have referred to him. He doesn't have to resort to aggressive salesmanship.

Nor should you fall into the trap of judging a doctor's competence by the amount of personal publicity he receives. A physician may project a charismatic image over the TV tube; he may possess a pleasingly resonant voice on radio; and he may have a talent for tossing out highly quotable remarks to the press. But these attributes are no guarantee that he performs at a high level in the operating room.

3. *Are you and the doctor compatible?* Just as in a marriage, compatibility is a key factor in a successful doctor-patient relationship. As a patient, you should look for a doctor who not only possesses the requisite skill but inspires comfort and confidence.

Maybe you're the type of patient who says to his doctor: "You're the doctor. Whatever you do is fine. Tell me what to do, and I'll do it." If so, you want a directive doctor — one who will give you a list of orders to follow. Or maybe you're exactly the opposite kind of patient. You wouldn't dream of accepting a course of treatment until the doctor explained in the greatest detail the whys and wherefores of what he had planned for you. If so, you'd be much happier with a doctor who enters into a participatory relationship with his patients. Matching doctors and patients allows treatment to proceed with a minimum of stress.

4. *Does the doctor have a trained staff to assist him?* Establish as diplomatically as you can whether or not the doctor is backed up by trained nursing assistants to help him perform the transplants.

I raise this question because hair transplanting involves a great deal of meticulous, detailed work — usually too much work for one person to do comfortably. But the doctor's helpers must know what they are doing. I was once invited to witness a hair transplant performed by a busy surgeon in a large U.S. city. I watched as he removed the plugs of hair from his patient and handed them over to his nurse for "cleaning." I noticed to my utter astonishment that her "cleaning" included snipping off the roots of many of the hairs. Naturally, there would later be little hair growth when the plug was transplanted to the bald spot. When I pointed this out to her, she was grateful, explaining: "All this stuff is new to me. I've only been working here for a week." Needless to say, this was an extreme case, but it provides an example of the potential problems associated with unqualified assistants.

In order to avoid this source of trouble, some surgeons do all the work themselves, including the cleaning of the plugs. One result is that such surgeons must increase their fees in order to cover this added use of their valuable time. There is no need for a physician to do the entire procedure himself, provided that he takes the time to train assistants adequately and that he retains their services after they've become experienced.

Here are a few additional tips:

1. Don't base your final choice on what the doctor charges for his services. At present, the going rate is $10 to $20 per plug in most centers. But as you travel from place to place, you'll notice a tremendous range in fees, varying from $1 to $50 per plug.

Most of the first-rate hair transplanting surgeons I know charge between $12 and $20 per plug. The man who charges more doesn't necessarily perform better, but at the other extreme, don't go looking for bargains. In most cases, you get what you pay for. Hair transplanting is expensive because you require a surgeon who possesses both medical expertise and artistry and because the surgeon will generally spend more time on you than he would to complete any other cosmetic procedure—four to eight operations, each of which will take 1½ to 4 hours.

2. Don't be impressed by a physician whose only apparent qualification is that he's been transplanting hair for a long time or that he has done thousands of operations (a favorite claim of advertisers). It's possible to go on repeating the same mistakes for five, ten, or even twenty years and for five, ten, or even twenty thousand operations.

3. In hair transplanting, as in other matters, distant pastures

sometimes look greener. Some patients will seek out surgeons who live 500 or 1,000 miles away, although there are practitioners of equal skill within a few miles of their homes. Other things being equal, you're better off in the hands of a doctor who lives and works in your area. He's more available to you; you're more available to him.

On the other hand, if after careful deliberation you find that the only suitable doctor lives out of town, then place yourself in his hands despite the added expense and inconvenience. After all, you've only got one head, and take my word for it, there's very little worse than a bad hair transplant.

4. Hair transplanting has become a fertile field for exploitation by the unscrupulous because of its growing acceptance by the public. I want to conclude this chapter, therefore, by repeating myself somewhat and warning you again about the various kinds of false advertising and misleading claims you may encounter.

For example, you may be favorably impressed by the surgeon you have interviewed as well as the photos he has shown you. But are you certain that he's the doctor who will operate on you? Are the photographs he's displayed samples of *his* work? In some "clinics," the actual transplanting is performed by a number of salaried physicians whose qualifications are not known to you. The photos you are viewing may be the handiwork of another doctor who works for the clinic.

Or you may go to a hair studio operated by a layman. You may be sold on a transplant with the understanding that the surgeon will be provided. Unfortunately, this leaves you with no way of checking on the competence of the man to whom you will entrust your health and appearance. All too often, the surgeon engaged by the studio is a recent medical graduate, at present a resident or an intern, whose main qualification is that he wants to earn a few extra dollars by moonlighting. A good rule of thumb is to insist on having the name, address, and phone number of the doctor who will operate on you, so that you can check on his credentials and experience.

You should be wary of transplants offered at "bargain" rates. Also watch out for low estimates of the number of grafts needed. The advertiser may deliberately underestimate the number of plugs required to restore your hair—hence the modest price. Later, he'll revise his estimate upward, and of course you'll have a lot more to pay.

Some operators may mislead you by using unnecessarily small plugs. It follows, therefore, that you'll require more plugs, and since you pay for each plug, there'll be a substantial increase in the total cost of your transplant.

You should be wary of ads that make liberal use of fancy and novel names to describe their hair replacement methods. The purpose is to suggest that you're being offered a unique and exclusive technique of hair replacement. You should be skeptical of such claims. Every first-rate physician makes it his business to keep abreast of the latest developments in his field. If there's a new way of restoring hair, your physician—if you chose him carefully—will know all about it. You can be certain that if a new technique is safe and an improvement over established methods, he'll make it available to you.

4

Are You a Good Candidate for Transplanting?

Let's assume that you've decided, on the basis of the information you've gathered, that you want a hair transplant and that you've selected a surgeon. That's a good start. You're ready for the next stage: an interview with him—which has two purposes.

First, your doctor will attempt to educate you and to allay your fears about hair transplant surgery by providing you with simple and direct answers about the procedure. He will tell you how much time you'll lose from work, how much the surgery will cost, how much pain you should expect, and so on. Your anxiety is completely natural. All of us feel threatened when faced with a surgical procedure about which we know little or nothing. The next chapter will cover the most common questions asked by patients, and the answers should go a long way toward satisfying any questions you have thought of.

The second purpose of the interview is to enable the physician to make a decision about you: Are you or are you not a suitable candidate for a transplant? Not all bald men can be helped by transplants, and the poor candidate should be firmly counseled against embarking on the procedure. This will save a lot of disappointment and recrimination later on.

Surgeons apply several criteria when assessing an applicant's suitability for a hair transplant. Although it is seldom possible to rate a candidate as "ideal," the number of bald men who can't be improved is relatively small. Your doctor will tell you how much he can do for you, and then you will have to decide whether that's enough to satisfy you and therefore whether or not it's worthwhile to proceed with transplanting.

The following are some of the more important guidelines that are used in judging an applicant:

Motivation and Expectations

Transplanting is a lengthy, drawn-out procedure, often requiring four or more sessions, spread out over at least several months. The patient, therefore, must not only be enthusiastic about the operation, but must also have the persistence and the determination to complete the course of treatment. The insufficiently motivated patient will lose interest after one or two sessions, and he'll end up with an incomplete transplant. If that happens, he will look worse after treatment than before.

We also dissuade applicants who are convinced that a bit more hair is all that stands between them and wealth, sexual abundance, social popularity, and all-round happiness. Like the forty-two-year-old salesman who blamed the loss of his last three jobs on baldness. (He had a drinking problem.) Or like the thirty-four-year-old professional who had just lost another girl friend because "my receded hairline makes me look old, and what young girl wants to be seen with an old man?" (He had a hostile, defensive manner that both men and women found unattractive.) We refer such people to a psychiatrist or a psychologist in the hope that they'll be helped to come to grips with their real problems.

Fortunately, most applicants are neither neurotic nor unrealistic in their expectations. They make modest demands. They want to roll the clock back a little — not back to the time when they had a bushy, teenage head of hair.

What kinds of men consult doctors about a hair transplant? A review of several hundred of our patients revealed the following:

They vary in age between seventeen and seventy years. Approximately 50 percent of them are blue- or white-collar workers. Among the other 50 percent, the largest professional group are doctors, followed by business executives and teachers.

There's a popular belief that men who seek hair transplant surgery are inordinately vain about their appearance. My own lengthy and firsthand experience in interviewing applicants has led me to a different conclusion. In a general way, they are no more vain than any other group of men. But they are different, inasmuch as they are particularly sensitive about going bald, and replacing the hair lost is a matter of importance to them. I find this neither unusual nor pathological. Many of us seem to give special importance to some aspect of our appearance or image, be it our teeth, our weight, the clothes we wear, or the car we drive. We gladly exchange money for the satisfaction of "feeling right." As I indicated earlier, most hair transplant patients are not wealthy. These patients can afford hair transplant surgery because they prefer to spend their money on improving their appearance rather than in acquiring a new car or a new wardrobe or in taking a trip abroad. They're convinced that with more hair they'll look better, they'll feel better, and that therefore they'll behave better.

Typical of my patients are the following:

A twenty-seven-year-old prematurely bald lawyer who was looking for a wife. He felt that he could improve his effectiveness as a suitor if he looked more like his real age, that is, if he had more hair.

A forty-five-year-old happily married major contractor who said simply: "There's no need to be bald anymore, so why should I be?"

A middle executive in publishing, age thirty-five, who was working in a highly competitive setting and was fearful that his receded hairline and bald crown were jeopardizing his chances for a promotion because his company was youth oriented.

A highly successful fifty-four-year-old president of a sales firm who was planning to resign and look for a new position in a slightly different field. He explained to me: "A bit of hair will knock five or ten years off my age, and that will give me a wider choice of jobs to choose from when I go looking. I know I'm good at my job—but if I'm turned down on the basis of my age, I won't have the opportunity to prove it."

All surgeons have had at least a few patients who were disappointed in the outcome of their transplants, and I'm no exception. But that's offset by the unbridled enthusiasm expressed by some patients over a very modest hair gain.

I'm thinking of the wealthy real estate man whom I turned down on three occasions. I explained to him that a hair transplant was not the solution to his problem because I couldn't possibly transplant enough hair over his vast bald area to make an appreciable difference in his appearance. He stubbornly refused to accept my decision. "Look," he said. "You've leveled with me, so your conscience should be clear. You don't think the operation should be done. I disagree with you. I know it won't make a huge difference in the way I look, but it will make some difference, and I'll be satisfied with that. My health is good, and I can easily afford your fee, so what can we lose? Please go ahead and operate."

I finally relented—on condition that he would first agree to a psychiatric consultation. Back came a report from the psychiatrist saying that the real estate man was normal in every respect; he just wanted a little more hair. I performed the transplant, and my patient was ecstatic about the results. I didn't share his enthusiasm, but I comforted myself with the thought that he got even more than he expected and was totally satisfied.

Age

There is no "best age" to transplant hair. Excellent results can be expected with patients from twenty-one to seventy years of age and older.

One might expect that an older individual with less efficient blood circulation to the scalp (due to the constriction of the blood vessels that occurs with age) would be a poor risk for a hair transplant. This is not so. Several of my best results have occurred with patients who were in their fifties and sixties. There is no arbitrary upper age limit for hair transplanting, provided that the person enjoys good health.

Applications from very young people are carefully scrutinized — and with good reason. A young man of eighteen or nineteen, for example, tends to be more anxious about premature hair loss and to act more impulsively in seeking a transplant. Later, he's more apt to become impatient and to drop treatment in midstream. Filling in recessions with transplants, for example, absolutely requires additional transplanting if and when hair is lost farther back — or else you end up with two unnatural-looking peninsulas of hair sticking out in an otherwise bald area. Once recessions are done, it isn't necessary to transplant the entire top of your head if it goes bald, but it is necessary to finish at least the front one-third if you don't want to look absurd. (This incidentally will frame your face and make you look your age instead of ten or fifteen years older.)

In addition, it's more difficult to predict with accuracy how large a young person's bald area will ultimately become. Planning becomes treacherous. You may take hair from an area that is destined for loss. Therefore, at the appointed time the hair will fall out at the site where it's been transplanted. The number of years that a person will retain any part of his hair is genetically programmed at the time of his birth, and one can only make an educated estimate, based primarily on his family history, of what the future holds. When dealing with young patients, therefore, we tend to underestimate the potential permanent donor area, allowing for a wide margin of safety. After five, ten, or fifteen years, one can always come back and do more transplanting if the size of the permanent rim is wider than was allowed for.

The Health Factor

Patients are not accepted unless they are in good health and can undergo the transplanting operation without risk.

We require all applicants for a transplant to see their own doctors for a complete physical examination within three months prior to starting surgery. We later check with the patient's physician and dentist, asking them if they know of any health reason that the transplant should not take place or whether there are any medical factors that we should be aware of. This procedure eliminates as completely as possible the chances that a patient has recently acquired a health problem or that he's forgotten something in his medical history.

Many surgeons do not require a complete preoperative physical examination. The fact that their patients come to no harm suggests that I may be too cautious — but in any case such an examination is probably a good idea for anyone who hasn't had one for a year or more, whether or not the person is contemplating surgery.

A complete history of a patient's medical background can be of practical value in many specific ways. A patient, for example — especially an older one — may have a history of minor vascular or heart disorders. This could result in a serious adverse reaction to some of the drugs we use while transplanting, epinephrine, for instance, which we employ to curb bleeding. But it also increases the blood pressure and stimulates the heart.

It's important to know in advance whether a person is a "bleeder," that is, someone whose blood clots with great difficulty and who therefore bleeds profusely when he's cut.

A history of allergy is obtained from the patient and his physician so as to minimize the chances of a potentially serious allergic reaction to any of the drugs we use before, during, and after surgery.

Finally, we watch for applicants who heal with hypertrophic scars or keloids, that is, patients whose surgical cuts don't heal in a smooth, natural way. Instead, they're left with an unsightly, bumpy ridge where the skin was broken. Blacks are more susceptible to hypertrophic scarring and keloids than are whites. If a keloid is found anywhere on an applicant's body, most physicians won't operate until they've performed a trial graft in an inconspicuous area of his head to see how well (or how poorly) it heals.

Don't automatically conclude that you're ineligible for a hair transplant because you suffer from any of the conditions I've mentioned above. Every case is judged on its own merits, and if deemed advisable, the operation is carried out by means of modified procedures. For example, if you're allergic to one drug, the doctor can substitute another. If you have a history of heart trouble, providing it's not too serious, you may be able to proceed with the transplant by scheduling multiple small sessions instead of a few large ones.

Hair Factors

Quantity.   Ideal patients have limited areas of baldness, such as the crown or the front one-third of the scalp. In such patients, sufficient donor sites are available to transplant the entire bald area solidly in four or more sessions and to obtain an excellent density of hair growth (Fig. 16A–16E in the color insert, and Fig. 17A–17E). Of course, the age of the patient and the prospects for the eventual enlargement of any areas of baldness must always be taken into consideration.

When larger areas of baldness are being treated, one must frequently accept the fact that there aren't enough donor grafts available to transplant the entire bald spot solidly. Therefore, some of the baldness must remain untreated. (Alopecia reduction, described in Chapter 2, is often useful in minimizing the size of this area.)

Alternatively, one can choose to use relatively dense transplanting in cosmetically strategic sites, such as the front hairline and the center of the crown, and only one, two, or three sessions over the rest of the scalp. Many patients prefer to spread about available grafts in this fashion rather than have dense hair growth in one area and no hair in another.

If less than four sessions are used in any given area, areas of baldness are inevitably left within the transplanted zone and the patient's scalp in that area will look somewhat like a "doll's head" on close inspection. The less dense the transplanting in any area, the greater the effort that must be put into hairstyling in order to create the illusion of a full head of hair. Don't try to cover too much with too little, or you will forever be combing, teasing, and spraying your hair down to make it look presentable. Your physician should tell you how much hairstyling will be required for whatever area objective you have chosen. Then you may or may not have to scale the objective down. If you and your doctor are not too ambitious, you can cover very sizable areas, and any tufting should be easily concealed with very little hairstyling (Figs. 23A–23G and 24A–24D).

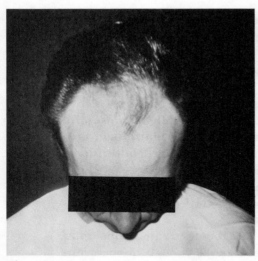

Fig. 17A. Before: (1) relatively small bald area, (2) reddish-brown hair, and (3) hair of moderately fine texture.

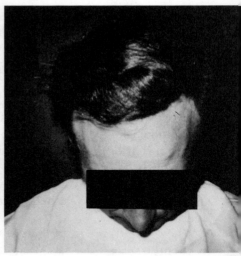

Fig. 17B. After—sixteen months after starti transplanting.

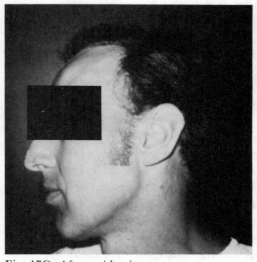

Fig. 17C. After—side view.

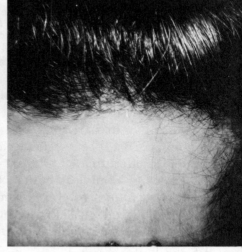

Fig. 17D. After. Hairline with hair comb up to expose it.

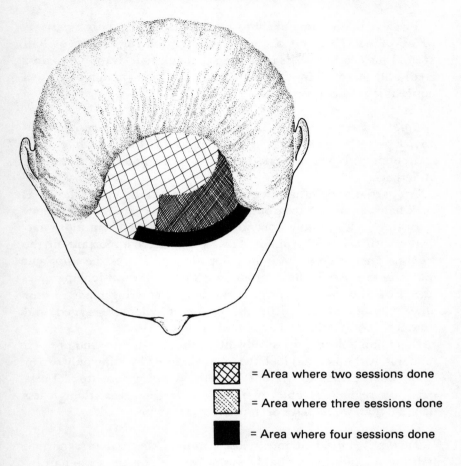

= Area where two sessions done

= Area where three sessions done

= Area where four sessions done

Fig. 17E. Five sessions, with a total of 350 grafts. (Done from 1973 to 1974, when smaller sessions were used than now.)

During the past four and a half years this patient has returned once or twice every one or two years for additional sessions to his mid-scalp and crown, keeping pace with thinning in these areas in such a way that nobody was aware that further transplanting was being done. (He had sufficient hair in the thinning areas at the time of surgery that it camouflaged the operations without difficulty.) Eventually, 692 grafts were done and we have transplanted the entire top of his scalp.

The candidate most likely to be rejected is one with a vast expanse of baldness and a correspondingly narrow fringe of hair around his head. There's simply not enough hair available to do a creditable job of filling in the bald spot, or even enough to make a noticeable cosmetic improvement.

Color.   Each physician has his own color preferences. Personally, I prefer to work with light-colored hair, that is, white, "salt and pepper," blond, or pale red—in approximately that order of preference.

I'm partial to light hair because it does not stand out as starkly as dark hair against a background of pale or pink skin. Any tendency to tufting or a thinning appearance therefore blends in more naturally with the background. This is especially important in the hairline area, where the light color also minimizes the apparent diameter of the hair shaft, producing a more natural-looking hairline. In addition, white or salt and pepper coloring tends to blur any abruptness of the hairline by making it look more ragged (and therefore more natural) than it actually is.

Light hair coloring is also advantageous for patients who prefer a moderately thinned-out look, which is achieved by using only two or three sessions instead of four sessions in any given area. These patients are thereby able to transplant larger areas (though less densely) than would have been possible otherwise.

Texture.   Fine hair most closely mimics the hair in a normal hairline. In addition, as baldness slowly develops, the scalp hair involved gradually becomes finer. As has been noted previously, the end result of hair transplanting is usually an "early thinning" appearance, and fine hair most closely mimics the natural state of the hair shafts at this stage in hair loss. Although the results in patients with fine hair do not appear as thick as some would prefer, they can be good enough to be virtually indistinguishable from the natural without very close inspection (See Figs. 10C and 10D, 17C and 17D. In the color insert, see Figs. 18B, and 47C and 47D.).

Patients who have "wiry" or "kinky" hair tend to have few fine hairs in their hairline, and the final results of transplanting are therefore not that unlike the original appearance (Figs. 21A–21D).

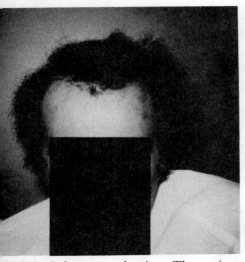

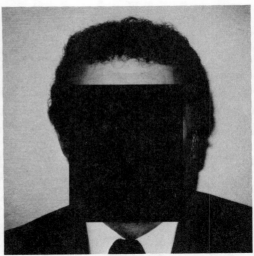

Fig. 21A. Before transplanting. The patient wanted his hairline moved forward about three inches. He had (1) very dense donor hair, (2) wiry textured hair with a natural curl, and (3) a small proposed recipient area.

Fig. 21B. After transplanting. Note the top crease on the patient's forehead in the "before" photo and in this one.

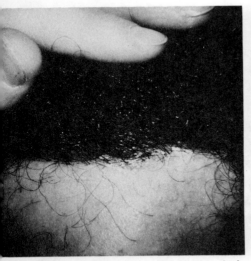

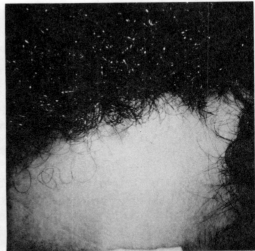

Fig. 21C. Transplanted hairline with hair lifted up to expose it.

Fig. 21D. Transplanted hairline lying naturally.

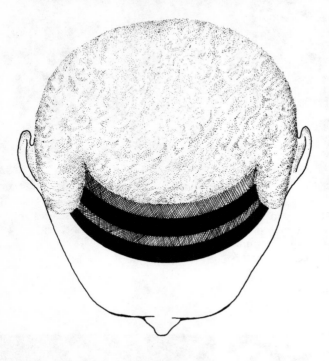

 = Area where three sessions done

 = Area where four sessions done

Fig. 21E. Four sessions, with a total of 325 grafts. Alternate bands of four and three sessions to produce a very thick-looking result with the hairstyle this patient had chosen.

Many of these patients also have a natural curl to their hair which (*a*) makes hair growth look thicker than it actually is; and (*b*) allows for a naturally curled hairline that completely disguises the coarse hair shafts.

Skin Coloring

Because the skin of the transplanted grafts has always been protected from sun exposure by overlying hair, it has never aged.

Therefore, when set in the forehead, these grafts may be conspicuous because of their paleness, compared to the adjacent skin. The paler your skin the better. The darker your skin, the greater the contrast will be and the more noticeable the color difference. There's a simple solution to this problem: Spend a lot of time out in the sun. Exposure of the grafts to the sun's rays will soon "age" the skin, and it will then blend into the coloring of the forehead after anywhere from a few months to several years (six to twelve months on average). Patients who achieve a blending of the old and new skin most readily are those with ruddy complexions or a Celtic background (redheaded, freckled, green-eyed ancestors) with easy-to-sunburn (easy-to-age) skin. Proper hairstyling (and in some cases make-up) can be used to camouflage the different coloring until nature and time does it for you.

5

What You Should Know about Hair Transplant Surgery: Common Questions and Answers

In this chapter, I want to provide brief answers to the questions patients most often ask about hair transplant surgery. Nearly all of the answers are covered elsewhere in the book, but the frequency with which these questions come up suggests that they warrant extra attention.

1. *How serious is hair transplant surgery?* It's regarded as minor surgery, and the likelihood of any serious consequences is extremely slight.

2. *Do hair transplants always work?* If the patient follows a few simple instructions and the doctor knows what he's doing, 100 percent of hair transplants "work." An *occasional* plug may not grow a good crop of hair—in which case it can be replaced—but virtually all grafts will "take," and there is no such thing as the unlucky person in whom transplanting just doesn't work.

3. *How much will the operation hurt me?* Believe it or not, it shouldn't hurt very much. Unfortunately, there is no single answer

that fits everyone, because what's "painless" to one patient can be "unbearable" to another. The best way for you to answer the question of your own "pain tolerance" is to ask yourself how much a visit to the dentist hurts you as compared to the comments of his other patients (for example your family).

On the other side of the equation is your doctor. Some physicians seem to be able to do some things a great deal less painfully than others doing supposedly the same thing — just as some dentists seem to hurt more than others. This can partly be explained by one physician having a "light hand" as compared to his colleagues but also it is related to how much effort your doctor actively puts into making the procedure less painful for you. For example, does he use premedication to allay fear and/or pain? Does he use very fine needles or routine ones? Does he use needleless injectors (explained later)? And does he use a good anesthetic technique (also explained later)? If you are a patient with an average pain threshold and he is one of those doctors who puts particular effort into making the procedure as comfortable as possible, you should find the whole operation roughly comparable to your dentist filling a cavity.

After the operation, and after the effect of the local anesthetic wears off (in 3 to 5 hours), there is usually only mild discomfort. In fact, as hard as it may be for you to believe, *most patients find it unnecessary to use any painkillers.*

If there is postoperative pain, all you need to do is call the doctor, and a pill can be prescribed to eliminate it. I tell my patients that any pain they have post-operatively is their fault. All they have to do is call and tell me they are having pain, and I will order the appropriate pill — usually Percodan or Demerol — to remove it. The only reason for them to have pain, therefore, is their reluctance to phone me. Don't be afraid to call your doctor if you are one of those who have significant discomfort. You shouldn't endure pain if you don't have to.

4. *How perfected is the hair transplanting procedure?*   Major advances have been made in the last five years or so. These include:

(a)   The ways of minimizing pain described in the previous question and in Chapter 6.

(b)   Much-improved operative technique.

(c) The incorporation of alopecia reduction into hair transplanting (discussed earlier in this book).

(d) More rapid removal of bandages and better postoperative
"cleanup," allowing earlier hair washing and hairstyling.

Although further improvements are no doubt inevitable, they
will probably be chiefly in the realm of making the procedure even
more comfortable rather than in improving the results significantly.

If you are one of those who had your transplant done 10 to 20
years ago you should think about a reassessment now. It might be
possible to significantly improve your results if you have any donors
left, and the operation will be much more pleasant than your
memories of it.

5. *Can transplanting ever produce completely natural
results?*   No. Regardless of how good a candidate you are, and of
how good your doctor is, the hair will never be distributed *perfectly*
evenly in the transplanted site. Parting through it will always reveal
some "tufting." On the other hand, the *illusion* of perfection should
be possible with little or no hair grooming effort, provided that you
and your doctor haven't tried to cover too much with too little (Figs.
22A–22E, 23A–23G, and 24A–24D).

6. *How much will the operation cost?*   That depends on how big
the bald area is, how much of it you want covered, how densely it
will be transplanted, and what your doctor charges per graft (plug).
(This is explained more fully elsewhere in the book.)

With few exceptions, physicians bill according to the number of
plugs they take from your fringe and transplant to your bald area.
Most reputable physicians charge between $10 and $20 per graft,
but the rate can vary below or above this price range, depending on
local conditions. The average bald patient is satisfied with transplanting the front one-third to one-half of his scalp and has 300 to
400 plugs done. The cost would therefore usually be somewhere between $3,000 and $8,000. The charge can be as little as $750, or, if
you want to cover a very large bald area, and/or if your doctor's fee
is higher than average, it can run from $7,500 to $15,000 or more.

7. *Will my health plan pay for my hair transplant?*   Unless the
hair loss was caused by accident or disease, health plans do not pay
for transplanting. However, if you are employed in certain
occupational categories—such as acting or modeling—and you can

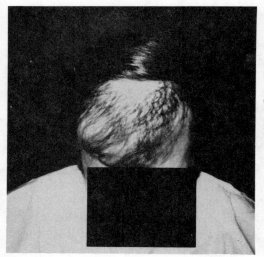

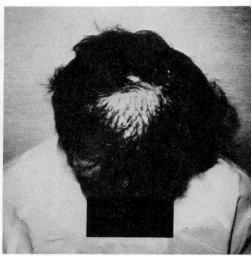

Fig. 22A. This man was virtually bald in the front one-third of his scalp prior to transplanting (he had a small tuft of hair left at the very front of his head). This photo, taken five months after he began treatment, shows small clumps of transplanted hair growing in a U shape behind the persisting tuft.

Fig. 22B. Eight and a half months after transplanting was begun, three sessions are growing in the U. A session was completed in the bald area behind the U six weeks before this photo was taken, and another session in the same zone has just been completed.

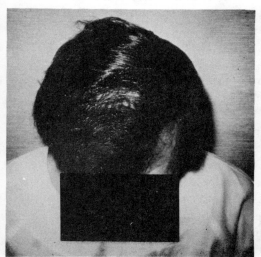

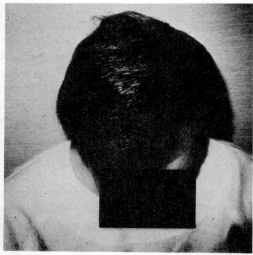

Fig. 22C. Twelve months after starting transplanting. Four sessions had been done in the U, and two had been done in the area behind the U (only one was growing at this point). A third session was done behind the U just after this photo was taken.

Fig. 22D. Appearance after sixteen months (500 grafts).

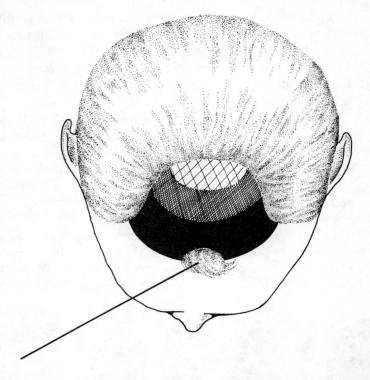

Tuft of persisting hair. Two sessions were done in this area for the present in order to thicken it and make it blend better with the thicker transplanted areas. Grafts have been saved to do two further sessions in this area whenever the rest of the original hair is lost (in pace with such loss).

The width of the four-session band is wider than that used in most patients. This patient is an actor and is filmed during "action shots" in wind, rain, etc. He therefore required thicker transplanting than most individuals would.

▨ = Area where two sessions done

▨ = Area where three sessions done

■ = Area where four sessions done

Fig. 22E. Seven sessions, with a total of 500 grafts.

show that hair transplant surgery was important in enabling you to earn your livelihood, you can claim the surgeon's fees as an income tax deduction. In addition, in most countries (including the United States), medical expenses are tax deductible whether or not they are incurred for cosmetic reasons and whether or not your appearance is important to your job. Check with an accountant.

8. *How many operations will I need?* This will be determined by the number of plugs that have to be transplanted and by the pattern that you and your doctor have chosen. The legends accompanying the photos in this book state the number of grafts that were done per patient and the number of sessions in which they were done. Some of the photos are also accompanied by schematic drawings of how the grafts were distributed. Hopefully, you will be able to get some idea of what you would need by reviewing those photos and finding one or more that show a bald area similar to yours and the final results you are hoping for. Most experienced doctors will do 75 to 100 grafts per session (which usually takes

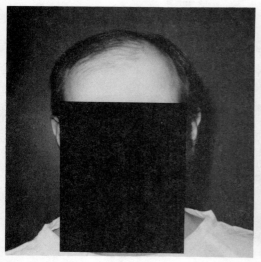

Fig. 23A. Before transplanting.

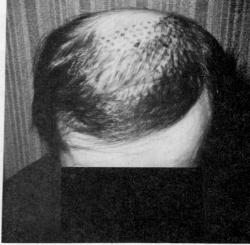

Fig. 23B. The growth of two sessions in the hairline area. A third session has healed and has just started to grow behind the front section on the man's left side. A fourth session is in the healing stage still farther back.

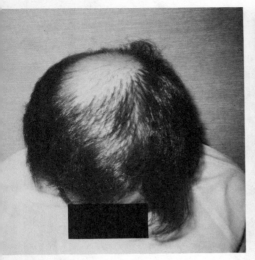

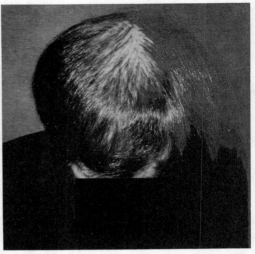

Fig. 23C. Three sessions are now growing in the hairline, and the fourth session, mentioned in Figure 23B, is also growing.

Fig. 23D. Fifteen months after starting transplanting. The hair has been parted through the midline to expose a "tufting" appearance in the mid-scalp. Solid transplanting was not done here so that a larger area could be covered.

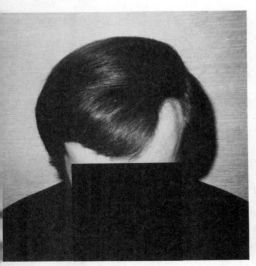

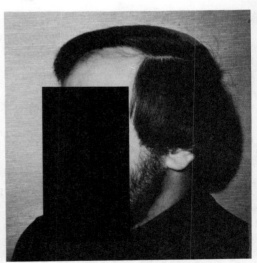

Fig. 23E. Hair transplanting completed and hair styled after fifteen months.

Fig. 23F. Side view at fifteen months.

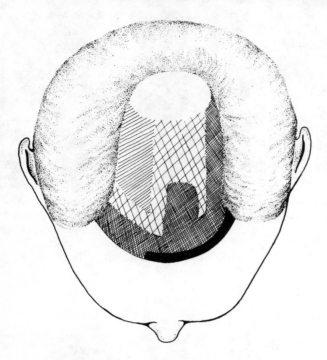

☐ = Area where zero sessions done

▨ = Area where one session done

▩ = Area where two sessions done

▦ = Area where three sessions done

■ = Area where four sessions done

Fig. 23G. Seven sessions, with a total of 560 grafts.

about two to three hours). If your baldness requires 400 plugs, you can count on having from four to six operations.

9. *How close together should the operations be?* The sessions have to be spaced out to allow each group of transplanted grafts to establish a good blood supply before the next group is done. Beware

of the practitioner who will "do it all" in one week or even in one or two months. If you rush from one operation to another, you can end up with less than optimal hair growth and a difficult-to-conceal clumpy-toothbrush appearance.

My approach is to do sessions of 75 to 120 grafts in any given area, and to allow six weeks between the first and second session, three to four months between the second and third session, and three to four months between the third and fourth session. Different areas of the scalp can be done in the intervals between these sessions—for example, the crown could be transplanted two days after an operation at the front of the head. The total treatment may therefore take 9½ months or more to complete.

Although there is usually a marked improvement in your appearance after one year, the full and final results of the transplant will not be seen for four to six months after that (Figs. 22D, 23D–23F, and 24B and 24C). By then the transplanted plugs will have blended into the rest of the skin and the hair will have reached a good length.

Some physicians do fewer grafts per session, proceed more quickly than I do (for example, forty to fifty grafts every three to six weeks), and produce good hair growth. I schedule long delays between my last two sessions for technical reasons that will be explained later, and I believe that this approach ultimately leads to better results in the cosmetically most important sites, i.e., the hairline and center of the whorl of the crown. However, it should be recognized that for some patients it's impractical to proceed slowly. You and your doctor may opt for what is most convenient for both of you. Small "repair" or "refinement" sessions may be done later to improve any imperfections in strategic areas such as the hairline.

10. *Can I expect to go bald again? How durable is transplanted hair?* Transplanted hair is very durable. We have records of such hair growing and thriving more than twenty years after it was grafted. There has never been a report in the medical literature of transplanted hair falling out. We expect transplanted hair to last as long as the hair in the fringe area from which it was taken. Most likely, that will be a lifetime.

11. *Will I have bald spots at the side and back of my head where the hair grafts have been taken?* Fortunately, this is not something

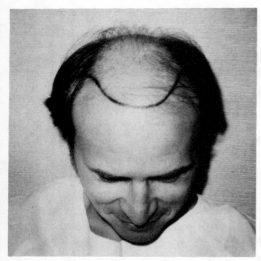

Fig. 24A. Before transplanting.

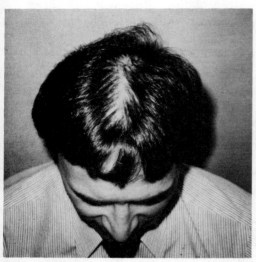

Fig. 24B. Sixteen months later, after transplanting, with the hair parted down the middle of the head. "Tufting" is present on the mid-scalp, where less than solid transplanting was done. If the transplanting had been done solidly throughout, a much smaller proportion of this patient's scalp would have been covered.

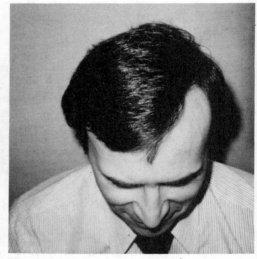

Fig. 24C. This photo was taken just after Figure 24B, but the hair is combed here as it is normally worn. This man does *not* need to use hair spray or other grooming arts to keep his hair in place. Transplanted hair is full enough to lie well on its own. (See also Figures 11A and 11B.)

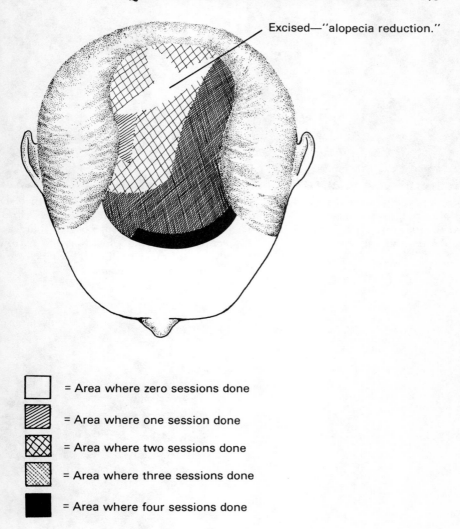

Fig. 24D. Ten sessions, with a total of 717 grafts.

you have to worry about. The circular punched-out areas do fill with hairless scar tissue, but it quickly shrinks until all that's usually left is a narrow line concealed by the hair surrounding it (Figs. 25A and 25B). The amount of scar shrinkage varies from person to person. If you are one of the unlucky few whose scars shrink very

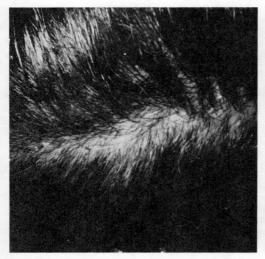

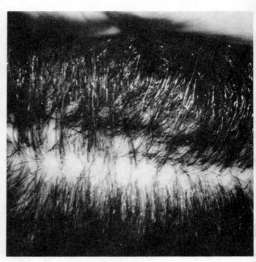

Fig. 25A. A properly harvested donor area six months after plugs were taken. Even with the hair parted this way, all that can be seen is an irregular narrow scar line.

Fig. 25B. A healed donor area that shows scar tissue. Plugs were taken too close together here, and the strip of hair that was left between rows and plugs was too narrow to allow for proper healing. This type of scar is unusual and unnecessary.

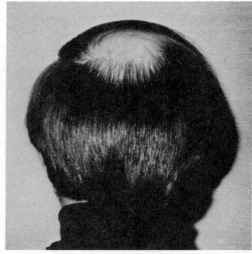

Fig. 26. This patient (the same one shown in Figure 23) had 560 plugs removed from the donor areas. Quite typically, there was virtually no change in the apparent density of hair growth.

little, your doctor will have to take fewer grafts than he could have otherwise. Without close inspection, your donor area should look essentially unchanged at the end of treatment (Fig. 26).

12. *Will I have a fairly good idea of what I will look like after my transplant is completed and all my hair is fully grown?*   Although one can't predict the outcome of every operation with complete accuracy, in most cases your doctor should be able to give you a fairly reasonable forecast of what you might expect.

13. *Can I transplant the whole bald area?*   The average patient can have 500 to 600 grafts removed (without any apparent change in hair density in the donor area). An occasional patient may have only 300 or fewer potential grafts (and may be rejected as a candidate for transplanting), while other patients may have over 800 potential grafts. If you have a large bald area, and therefore a correspondingly small fringe of hair, there won't be a large enough supply of hair in the donor site to cover all that baldness. Compromises will have to be made. You'll have to decide, with the help of your doctor, how the available hair can be deployed to achieve the best coverage. The usual method is a greater concentration of hair grafts toward the front section of your head and on the side where the part is. This enables you to comb thicker hair across the less densely transplanted area (Figs. 22A–22E, 23A–23G, 24A–24D, and 27A–27C).

If you have a small bald area—for example, only the crown or the front third of your scalp, or possibly even both—you should be able to transplant the entire bald area virtually solidly.

14. *Where should the hairline be?*   This is one of the most important decisions you will have to make. You can't have a successful hair transplant without a pleasing hairline. Indeed, as has been mentioned earlier, you can judge the skill and artistry of the hair transplant surgeon by the quality of the hairlines he constructs.

Select the height on your forehead where you want your hair to fall to, and then have the grafts implanted about one or two inches higher (Fig. 28). When you have hair again, it will naturally fall forward that distance (Figs. 29A and 29B). If you don't take this factor into account in advance, you may be stuck with a ridiculously low hairline.

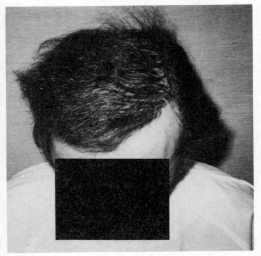

Fig. 27A. This patient had been bald on the front two-thirds of his scalp. Five sessions (384 plugs) had been done, and two more were scheduled in order to complete the original plan. Plugs had been placed more densely on the patient's left side (the part side) and more sparsely on the right, as the bald area was large and there weren't enough donor plugs to solidly transplant the entire bald zone.

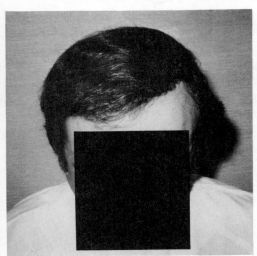

Fig. 27B. By parting his hair one and a half inches to two inches below the transplanted area and combing this hair across his head, the patient was able to make the uncompleted area look quite thick. Enough hair had been transplanted to prevent the hair from flying away in the wind. The patient decided that this situation was good enough and that he didn't need any more transplanting. I do not prefer this subterfuge, but unfortunately many patients do, and parting the hair lower allows them to employ it credibly.

Never try to move the front of your temples forward. The hair at this site is normally very fine and very sparse. A transplant is too thick and always looks artificial here.

If you have a large bald area and want to cover as much of it as

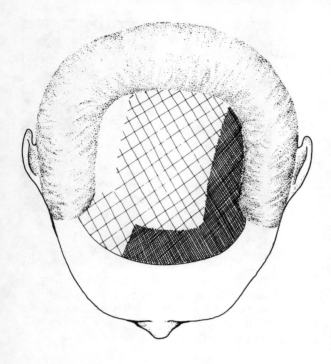

☐ = Area where zero sessions done

▨ = Area where two sessions done

▧ = Area where three sessions done

Fig. 27C. Five sessions, with a total of 384 grafts.

possible, keep in mind that the farther forward you choose the hairline, the more grafts you will need to transplant the front of the scalp and the less donor hair you'll have left to cover the bare areas farther back. (Moving a hairline forward only 3.0 to 3.5 millimeters

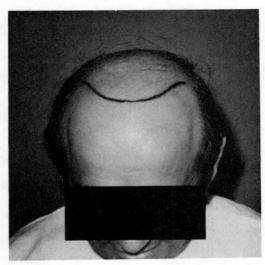

Fig. 28. New hairline marked in, keeping in mind that the new hair will fall forward one to two inches. The hairline is also slightly asymmetrical toward the part line, which will be on this patient's left side.

can require up to fifty plugs.) It is particularly important to remember this if you are young. Who knows exactly what the future holds for you? Perhaps you will develop a new bald area later in your life. If you have chosen a very low hairline and have expended a great number of plugs on it, there may not be enough plugs left in your donor area to cover the new bald zone. It is always wise to keep a few plugs "in the bank" for the future.

Lastly, a low hairline may be very becoming on a young man, but as you get older it fits in less and less naturally with the rest of your appearance. For all of these reasons, it's wise to choose a hairline that is as high as you can possibly accept.

15. *To what extent will the operation limit my activities?* This depends on what your normal activities are. If you're engaged in sedentary work, there's no reason why you can't go directly to your job from the doctor's office, provided, of course, that you are not self-conscious about the turbanlike bandage you have to keep on your head for twenty-four hours following the operation.

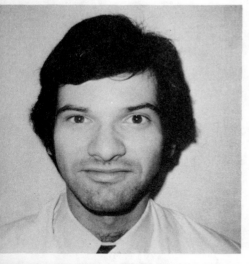

Fig. 29A. This young man's hair falls forward naturally quite far over his forehead.

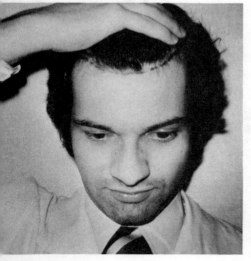

Fig. 29B. When the young man pulls his hair up, you can see how high his hairline really is—two to three inches higher than you might have guessed from Figure 29A. Keep in mind that when you have hair again, it too will tend to fall forward. If you don't take this factor into account in advance, you'll be stuck with a ridiculously low hairline.

For the first few nights, it's helpful to sleep propped up on pillows. This prevents or reduces postoperative swelling.

For a week after the operation, you should not engage in strenuous physical activities that cause an elevation in blood pressure, extra warmth, or perspiration. These factors may cause

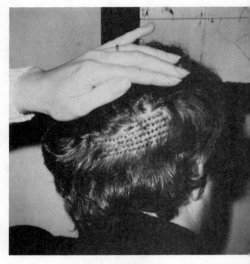

Fig. 30A. Donor site one week after the transplant operation.

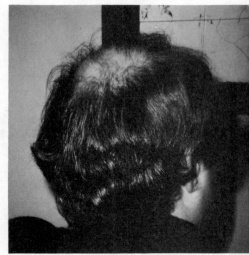

Fig. 30B. The donor site can be completely concealed immediately after the transplant operation by combing surrounding hair over it.

the plugs to loosen and pop out, and in addition they invite infection. It's also wise to go easy on your sex life during the first week.

16. *How will I look after the operation?* It's nearly always possible to conceal the signs of surgery in the donor site immediately

after the operation by combing hair over it (Figs. 30A and 30B). In twenty-four hours to three weeks you may be able to do the same in the recipient area, depending on how large the area is and how much hair you had left before you started transplanting (Figs. 14A and 14B). The plugs will have small crusts on them for one to three weeks after each operation.

Some patients prefer to wear a hairpiece during the course of treatment. Although many physicians allow a hairpiece within twenty-four hours of the operation, some (including me) prefer that a hairpiece not be worn during the first week after each session and that it be worn as little as possible during the second week. The warmth and moisture underneath hairpieces are conducive to infection, so that it is probably wisest to avoid them during this initial period.

17. *How should I prepare myself for the operation?* Get a good night's sleep. If you live in another city, it's wise to check into a hotel near your doctor's office the night before surgery.

Eat moderately. The possibility of becoming nauseated during surgery is increased if you've overindulged, whereas the likelihood of feeling faint during surgery is increased if you haven't eaten enough. Keep away from aspirin and vitamin E (for one and two weeks, respectively) before the operation, and from alcohol for twenty-four hours. These three substances tend to increase bleeding during and sometimes after the operation. Alcohol may also combine with the drugs used in surgery to produce unwanted and sometimes dangerous side effects. For the same reason, abstain from medications of all kinds before coming to the office. If there's a medicine you absolutely can't do without, discuss the matter with your doctor.

Shampoo your hair the night before or the morning of the surgery (you won't be able to wash it again for two to three days), but don't cut it. The longer your hair, the more effectively it can be used later to camouflage the areas operated on. If any hair trimming is needed, your doctor can take care of it just before the operation.

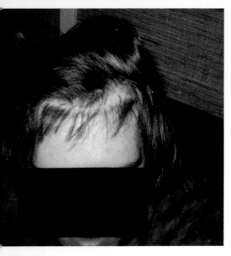

Fig. 8. This patient had a "free" strip graft placed across the front of his receding hairline. The hair in the strip was directed forward, and it would lie flat against his forehead, producing a "bang" effect. His hair was difficult to style in any other way. (A few poor punch grafts were also done by the same surgeon in front of and behind the strip.)

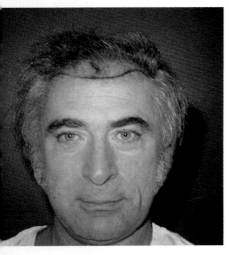

Fig. 16A. Before. This patient had (1) a relatively small bald area; (2) coarse, kinky hair; and (3) salt and pepper hair coloring. Moreover, (4) he was old enough that there was less need to "save" so many donor plugs for areas that might go bald in the future.

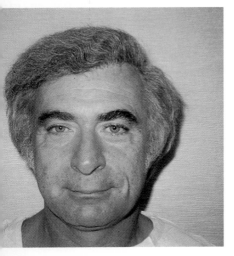

Fig. 16B. Fourteen months after transplanting was started (313 plugs in four sessions).

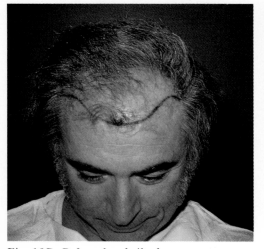

Fig. 16C. Before, head tilted.

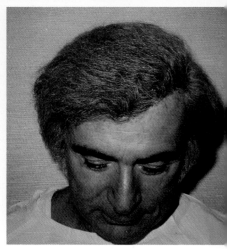

Fig. 16D. After. Subsequent to this pho
additional 135 grafts were done to fu
thicken this area and to "shore up" thir
areas behind the originally transplanted

Permanent rim

Thinning but still reasonable amount o'
when transplanting originally bega
1974. This area gradually thinned fu
and two years later another seventy
were placed here. In 1977 an addit
sixty-five grafts were done in this area
a third session was done to the zone o
sessions noted in this drawing. (Touch
in the hairline and elsewhere were do
the same time.)

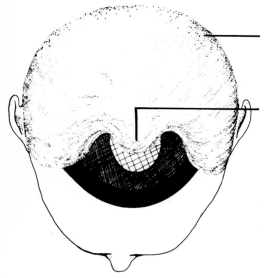

▨ = Area where two sessions done

▩ = Area where three sessions don

■ = Area where four sessions done

Fig. 16E. Four sessions, with a total of 313
grafts.

A total of 135 grafts have been done since the "after" photos shown in 16B
and 16D in order to keep pace with additional hair loss behind the original
bald area. (One further session in parts of this thinning area will probably
be necessary as more of his original hair is lost.) Neither of these two
"keeping pace" sessions were necessary, if the patient had been content with
going bald behind the transplanted area. Because they were done while there
was still some hair left in the site (to camouflage the surgery) nobody was
aware of them.

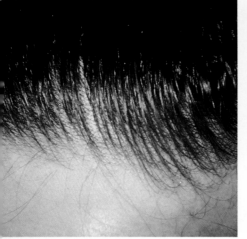

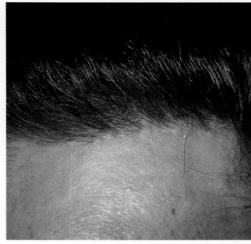

g. 18A. A normal hairline.

Fig. 18B. Transplanted hairline—fine hair.

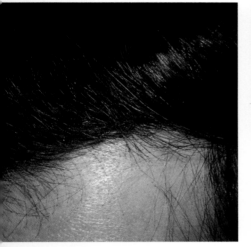

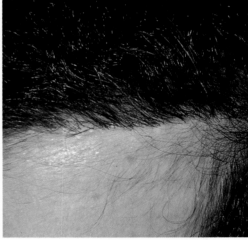

g. 19. Transplanted hairline—medium texture.

Fig. 20. Transplanted hairline—coarse texture.

More than the quality of the hair is involved in producing results similar to those shown above. Hair density in the donor area, hair coloring, how well the patient heals, skin coloring, and the physician's skill and artistry all play a role. Results like those shown above are not possible in all patients but demonstrate the potential of hair transplanting if there are enough positive factors present.

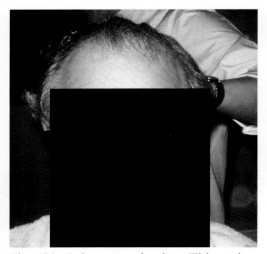

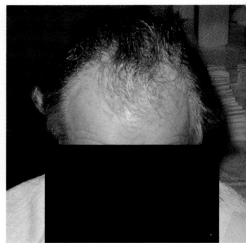

Fig. 47A. Before transplanting. This patient wanted his hairline moved forward approximately three inches and his central tuft thickened.

Fig. 47B. Before transplanting, with hea tipped slightly.

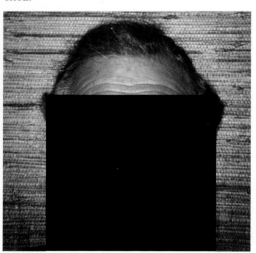

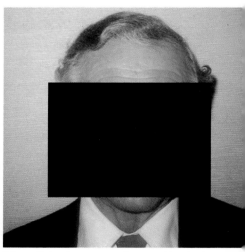

Fig. 47C. After transplanting. The initial growth was dense and far wirier than the hair·in the donor area from which it was taken. This wiriness is a temporary "shock reaction" that is seen in some patients. Three sessions (290 plugs) had been done. The usual fourth session was felt to be unnecessary.

Fig. 47D. One year later, all of the tran planted hair had regained its natural texture

6

The Operation:
What Happens during
the Transplant

In this chapter, I will try to give you a step-by-step description of what your transplant operation may be like. Although the fundamental procedures of a transplant are fairly standard, individual doctors have their own adaptations or variations of the technique. Therefore, your doctor will probably depart somewhat from the procedures described here. In a book of this kind, it's not possible to include all the alternative approaches currently in use.

Let's begin the day of your operation at 8:00 A.M., the time of your arrival at the office.

8:00 A.M.: *Presedation.* To lessen your anxiety, you will be given a tranquilizing drug. Because it takes a little time for the drug to act, you'll receive it about thirty to forty-five minutes before your surgery is scheduled. The most commonly used tranquilizing drugs are Valium and Demerol.

Valium is one of the world's most popular tranquilizers, and it has been for many years. It is usually given in pill form, and a fifteen-milligram dose will completely relax the average patient. Moreover, Valium has these added advantages: (1) It possesses painkilling qualities that will lessen the discomfort caused by the administration of injections during the operation. (2) It helps prevent or lessen the side effects that might be caused by large doses of anesthetic.

Demerol, a synthetic narcotic and a powerful painkiller, can be used with, or instead of, Valium. As a side effect, Demerol tranquilizes.

On occasion, for a specific reason, your doctor may decide to inject Valium or Demerol into your veins immediately prior to surgery, rather than have you swallow the drug in pill form. The patient reacts more quickly and more profoundly to the drug when it is administered intravenously than when it is taken by mouth. On the other hand, the intravenous route slightly increases the risks of adverse side effects.

A third drug, atropine sulfate, is sometimes used for patients who are extremely nervous or who have a history of fainting easily in a doctor's or dentist's office. Atropine has a chemical effect on your nervous system that counteracts the tendency to faint. Few individuals require atropine, and it is therefore not used routinely in hair transplant surgery. You or your doctor may decide to forgo Valium and Demerol because, for example, using them will make you unable to drive yourself home afterward.

8:30 A.M.: *Review of Plan and Preparation.*   Properly sedated, you walk into the treatment room and exchange your shirt for a gown.

You sit down on a chair in front of a mirror. You review the procedure agreed on at an earlier consultation, and the proposed hairline is drawn on your scalp. It's extremely important that the patient know exactly what his new hair pattern is going to be like in order to avoid disappointments and recrimination later on.

You may notice that the doctor is not working alone. Transplant surgeons are usually assisted by one or more nurses who are trained technicians in hair transplanting. They will help with the operation; "clean," prepare, and classify the hair plugs; and perform other tasks. This leaves the doctor free to concentrate on

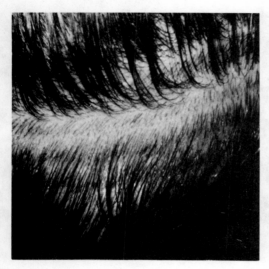

Fig. 31. Hair in the donor area is clipped to a length of one-eighth to one-fourth inch in lines separated by rows of intact hair one-fourth to three-eighths inch wide. These intact rows allow for better coverage of the donor area after the transplant operation. The site is then prepared with alcohol and another anti-bacterial solution. The direction of hair growth is clear, and it is followed when the plugs are punched out.

the surgery and on the selection of appropriate plugs for various sites.

A doctor who is well staffed can work faster. A procedure that can be completed in three hours with assistants could take five to eight hours without them. This extra time can be a strain on the patient. It can also result in a substantial increase in the doctor's fee.

The hair in the donor area is now clipped close to the scalp, but about one-fourth inch of hair is left to indicate the direction in which the hair is growing. Narrow rows of intact hair are also left between the clipped rows (to aid in post-operative camouflaging of the area). (Fig. 31). Next, the donor area and the recipient area are cleaned with alcohol. As an extra safeguard against infection, they are usually painted or sprayed with an antibacterial solution as well.

8:45 A.M.: *Anesthesia.*   You are lying on the operating table. Most doctors, myself included, prefer the prone to the sitting position during surgery because patients usually find it more comfortable and because fainting (or syncope) is less likely to occur if the patient is lying down. Fainting is rare, but it is a complication that

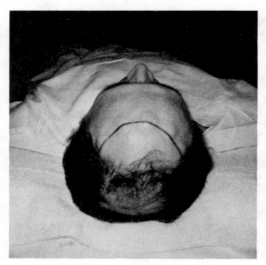

Fig. 32. Using a very fine needle (about the size of an acupuncture needle), five areas were frozen just in front of the proposed hairline (marked in black). After several minutes, a total "field block" was established painlessly by filling the gaps in the line of anesthesia from areas already frozen. After three to five minutes, any needles or surgery behind such a line will be painless.

should be avoided if possible. When it occurs, it worries patient and doctor alike. Although fainting isn't a serious problem, it can be confused with an adverse reaction to one of the drugs being used.

A few surgeons favor having the patient sit up because they feel that this gives them better access to the areas being operated on or because they find it easier to control bleeding when the patient is sitting up. I have operated on patients both ways: sitting up and lying down. With experience, access is not a problem (except occasionally in the crown area, in which case the patient can sit for part of the procedure) and with good assistants, bleeding can be well controlled regardless of the patient's position. Depending on the physician, his office set-up, and his staff, you may or may not be lying down, but I would advise you to opt for the lying position if you are given a choice, i.e., if your doctor is comfortable working with you either way.

The time has now come to administer the local anesthetic, or "freezing" solution. This prevents pain in very much the same way as freezing your gums prevents pain when your dentist works on your teeth.

Let me give you a brief lesson in anesthesia so you'll understand a

strategy that can afford you the greatest protection against unnecessary discomfort.

There are two basic things to grasp. First, the nerve supply to the
front of the head comes from the forehead, and the nerve supply to
the rest of the head comes up from the neck. Second, if you make a
series of freezing injections in a line across the forehead, you effectively block off any sensation of pain above that line (which is the
front of your scalp, or the recipient area) (Fig. 32). Similarly,
another series of freezing injections in a line on the nape below the
donor area cuts off all pain above that line.

This technique of blocking off pain to an entire area by injecting
the anesthetic at strategic points is referred to by physicians as a
"field" nerve block. In the course of the operation, it's necessary to
make dozens of anesthetizing injections. Thanks to the field nerve
block, however, the patient will feel pain only from the first few
injections. As was mentioned earlier, most of our patients say that a
transplant hurts only as much as or less than a visit to the dentist.
Most people find this very hard to believe. From the preceding, you
may understand how it is possible.

To further minimize the amount of pain you feel, your doctor
can give injections with an extremely fine needle ("thirty gauge"),
about the size of an acupuncture needle. Or he may dispense with a
needle altogether, and work with special instruments that can
propel liquids into your skin. This still stings a bit—but only
momentarily. Lastly, patients who have had "laughing gas" (nitrous
oxide) at the dentist's, and have tolerated it well, can be given it
prior to freezing—in which case they won't care about or feel any
pain. Some doctors are equipped to administer nitrous oxide;
others aren't. Check first if you want it.

8:50 A.M.: *Taking Grafts from the Donor Area.*   You are lying,
face down, on the operating table. Your anesthetized areas feel
somewhat like blocks of wood. The doctor now begins taking out
grafts from the donor area.

During a typical session, he will harvest four parallel rows of
grafts, each containing 20 to 25 plugs, or a total of 80 to 100 grafts.
However, depending on the needs of the individual patient—and

the preferences of your physician—as few as 20 plugs or as many as 150 may be transplanted at a single session.

The plugs punched out are usually four millimeters in diameter (that is, just over one-fourth inch), though some doctors prefer 4.5-millimeter grafts. In later sessions, the sizes of the grafts are varied to fit the sizes of the remaining spaces.

In taking grafts from the donor area, the doctor leaves about one millimeter between the plugs on any given row and a strip of intact hair about two to three millimeters in width between rows. There's a good reason for this spacing: If the plugs removed are too close to each other, healing is slower and the scars on the donor site may be more noticeable than they need be (Fig. 25B).

The instrument used to cut out the grafts in the donor area may be either a hand-driven "punch," which resembles a short metal drinking straw with a sharp end (Fig. 33A), or a power-driven machine which rapidly whirls a similar "punch" in a clockwise direction (Fig. 33B). I prefer the power punch. When applied to the scalp with only a slight amount of pressure, it bores out a plug in very much the same way as a cookie cutter punches cookies out of dough.

My preference is based on the fact that the power tool considerably reduces the sensation of pressure felt by the patient as the grafts are being cut. The newer models are virtually noiseless, and almost all of the patients whom I have treated with both types of instrument prefer the power model. Contrary to popular belief, using a power tool instead of a hand tool does not reduce bleeding or the pain that the patient experiences. There is no pain either way if the freezing has been done properly. Nor does the power tool enable the doctor to take more or better grafts. It simply makes hair transplant surgery easier for both the patient and his surgeon.

Some bleeding is inevitable when grafts are being taken from the donor site. Usually simple pressure by the doctor and his assistant is enough to stop it. If any site bleeds more than normally, the bleeding can be staunched by placing a coagulating pellet in the hole or, sometimes, by putting a stitch through it. (Such stitches are removed five to seven days later.) By the time all the grafts have been removed from the donor site, the bleeding should have been brought under complete control.

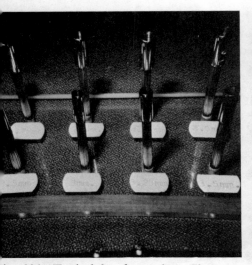

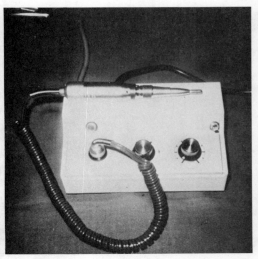

ig. 33A. Typical hand punches. These are ollow, strawlike cylinders with sharp cut-ng edges. Many different types and sizes are vailable.

Fig. 33B. A typical power punch. The entire unit is about the size of a standard telephone. Punches of various sizes are inserted into the small end of the metal barrel. They revolve clockwise when the instrument is turned on.

A few surgeons routinely stitch all the donor holes, whether or not these stop bleeding on their own. They claim that this prevents any chance of postoperative bleeding and makes the donor area easier to conceal—both of which it does. On the other hand, the more sutures, the tighter and sorer your scalp will feel when the freezing wears off an hour or two later. Sutures also increase the chances of postoperative infection in the donor area (though it would still be very unusual). Unless more than 100 to 120 grafts have been removed, camouflaging your donor area after the operation should not be a problem with or without suturing. Similarly, postoperative bleeding is rare (a fraction of 1 percent in my practice, for example) if proper precautions are taken during the operation. Suturing also causes some inconvenience if routinely used, as you will have to come back to have them removed. ("Self-dissolving" sutures take 1 to 2 weeks to dissolve and increase the possibility of infection). Consequently, many of us prefer to use a minimum amount of suturing unless patients have had problems with bleeding on prior occasions or are having very large sessions. It all boils down to weighing advantages over disadvantages, and different doctors and patients will come to different conclusions.

The next phase of the procedure — preparing the grafts for planting in the bald spot — is crucial. If the plugs are mishandled in any way, your hair transplant will not be wholly successful.

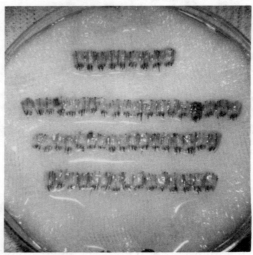

Fig. 34. After the grafts are cleaned, they are placed in a petri dish filled with a salt solution and arranged in rows according to the coarseness of the hair and the number of hairs per graft.

The plugs that have been removed consist of a tuft of hair embedded in skin that rests on a layer of fat. Working with great care the nurse or doctor clips away the excess fat, but leaves the hair roots intact. Leaving too much fat on the plugs can cause irritation after transplanting. On the other hand, trying to get *all* the fat off may accidentally injure the hair roots. The nurse also removes hairs without roots from the plugs. These hairs won't grow, and furthermore, if transplanted, they could be the site of future inflammation or infection. Lastly, any portion of the graft that does not contain hair — hair is sometimes distributed unevenly across the surface of a graft — is clipped away.

Once cleaned and trimmed, the plugs are placed in a glass, gauze-lined saucer that is filled with a salt solution to keep the plugs moist. The plugs are arranged in rows, according to the coarseness of the hair and the number of hairs per graft (Fig. 34). As you shall see shortly, there's a reason for this: One of the keys to a successful transplant is to place the right graft in the right place.

9:10 A.M.: *Preparing the Recipient Area.*   The doctor now begins to punch out a series of holes in the bald area into which the plugs will be planted.

If the bald recipient area is on your crown or the top of your head, you remain on your stomach. If it's on the front of your scalp, you turn over on your back to make the site of the operation more accessible. The head of the operating table is then raised to an angle of about forty-five degrees.

To ensure a snug fit, the recipient holes are made with a punch that is a little smaller than the one used to obtain the hair plugs. There's a reason for this: Hair grafts shrink a bit after they're removed from the scalp. At the same time, the holes made in the recipient area usually expand slightly. Thus, unless the recipient holes were made with a smaller punch than that used in the donor area they would be too large for the plugs and the patient would be left with a circular hairless scar around each graft. The correct difference in the size of the punches used in the donor and recipient areas varies from person to person, so no general rules for "differentials" in punch sizes are possible. Normally, we drill out the first recipient hole with a punch one millimeter smaller than that used in the donor area and then try one of the donor grafts in it to see whether the fit is right or too snug. If the fit is too tight, the hole can be enlarged with a slightly larger punch, and the graft tried again. This is repeated until the optimum differential for a patient has been established. The rest of the holes in the recipient area can then be made with the same-sized punch.

9:40 A.M.   The holes in the recipient area are completed. At this point, you'll be given a coffee break while the nurses finish cleaning and double-checking the plugs.

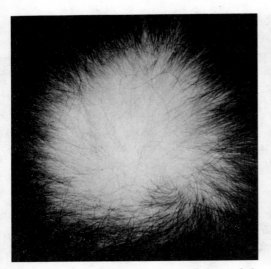

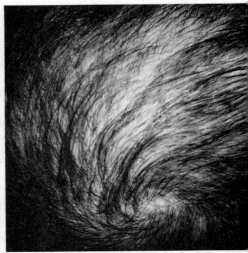

Fig. 35A. Before. The fine remaining adult hairs and vellus hairs shown here provided a "pattern" of the natural direction of this patient's hair growth.

Fig. 35B. The hair transplanted in the firs two sessions is growing, and the hair trans planted in the third session is just beginnin to grow.

9:50 A.M.: *Planting the Plugs in the Bald Area.*   Now begins the final phase of transplanting—inserting the hair-bearing plugs into the punched-out sites on the bald scalp. This is another crucial part of the procedure that must be performed with the utmost care.

First, any blood clots that may be present are removed from the bottom of the recipient holes. This enables the plugs to fit flatly and firmly in the scalp. It also ensures better nourishment for the newly planted grafts, since clots may interfere with the circulation of blood to them.

Appropriate plugs are now placed in the various recipient sites, beginning with the hairline, if that is the part being operated on, or with the center of the crown, if that is the recipient area. The plugs are then rotated so that the grafted hair is growing in the same direction as the original hair (Figs. 35A–35C and 36). To ascertain the growth direction of the original hair (if it is "totally gone"), the doctor inspects the scalp for fine hairs, known as vellus hairs. Even a "totally bald" person has a few vellus hairs left, and these provide

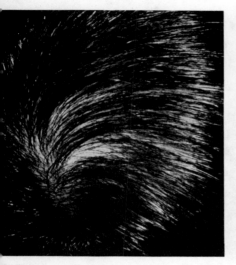

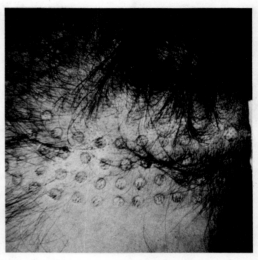

35C. After four sessions (375 plugs) and
een months.

Fig. 36. Grafts have been rotated so that the direction of hair growth follows the "pattern" provided by the remaining fine adult and vellus hairs.

the "pattern" information that the doctor needs to reproduce your original appearance.

Each plug insertion is carefully scrutinized to make sure that no adjacent hairs are accidentally trapped beneath it. A trapped hair can cause irritation or infection at some future time.

As I've stated throughout this book, the caliber of a hair transplant surgeon can be judged by looking at the quality of the hairlines he constructs. Mistakes made in the hairline are clearly visible, and the errors are usually difficult — and sometimes impossible — to conceal or correct without resorting to troublesome hairstyling or hair grooming techniques.

Your doctor will strive for a natural-looking hairline, that is, for a hairline composed of a moderately spaced growth of fine hair arranged in a ragged or random fashion and becoming gradually coarser and denser as one moves toward the back of the head (Figs. 37A and 37B). Therefore, the plugs for the front row of the hairline should not be placed in a straight row and they should ideally con-

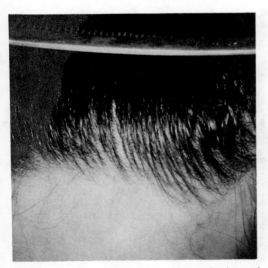

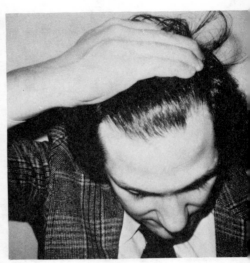

Fig. 37A. A natural hairline. Note the jagged front line, the moderately spaced fine hairs, the gradual increase in the coarseness of the hair as one goes farther back, and the hairs angling forward but combed back.

Fig. 37B. A more distant view of a natural hairline.

tain fine hair with a density of approximately twelve to sixteen hairs per plug. Plugs with coarser hairs and greater hair density (if available) could be used for the second, third, and fourth rows.

In addition, the best plugs are always used on the "part" side of the scalp, so that when hair grows it can be used to comb over the sparser "nonpart" side.

10:30 A.M.: *Bandaging.*   The surgical portion of the operation is now over, and you are ready for bandaging.

The underside of a nonsticking surgical dressing is spread with an antibiotic ointment and placed carefully over the transplanted grafts so as not to alter their position. The pad is then taped to the forehead or the crown of the head to prevent it from sliding, and gauze is packed over it.

The donor area is covered with a mixture of antibiotic ointment, and/or a coagulating powder (a powder that encourages blood clotting) or mesh and gauze pads are laid over it as well.

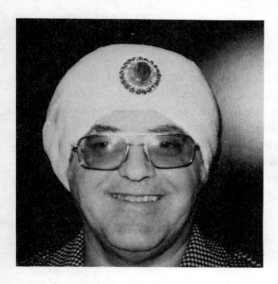

Fig. 38. A turbanlike "pressure bandage" is worn for twenty-four hours after the transplant operation. It prevents bleeding and accidental movement of the grafts from their proper position. This patient brought one of his wife's brooches as an added decorative touch.

Next, the entire head is wrapped in a white gauze "pressure bandage," which resembles a turban (Fig. 38). It's bound with enough pressure to keep the grafts firmly in place and properly orientated, and to minimize bleeding. For reasons of efficiency, the turban bandage covers the ears — a feature that may cause some discomfort. To minimize the chances of discomfort, the ears can be padded with cotton batting. If you find the pressure on your ears uncomfortable, you can loosen the bandage slightly after you get home by slitting it with scissors, just in front of the ear. A strip of adhesive tape across the slit will keep it from getting any larger and causing the bandage to become too loose.

At 10:45 A.M., your first session is over, less than three hours from the time you arrived at the office.

Some patients go directly from the session to their place of work. Patients who feel self-conscious about having the head swathed in a prominent bandage may take a few days away from their jobs. For the first operation — as I've mentioned earlier — I advise a week's holiday.

It's wise to err on the side of caution and avoid driving your car immediately following the operation. As you may recall, I noted above that some of the drugs used in the operation may temporarily impair judgment and coordination, so why take a chance? In particular, it's been shown that 15 milligrams of Valium can significantly alter driving ability for up to five hours after it's been taken, despite the fact that you may "feel" perfectly normal. If you happened to get into an accident, you could be legally charged with driving while under the influence of drugs.

Some of you will find the preceding description of the operation more detailed than necessary. Others will crave more information. If you are one of the latter group, I would suggest that you go to a medical library or a university bookstore and obtain one of the following medical references:

1. S. Ayres III. "Hair Transplantation." In Epstein, Ervin, *Skin Surgery,* 4th edition. Springfield, Ill.: Charles C Thomas, 1977.
2. W. P. Unger. *Hair Transplantation.* New York, Basel: Marcel Dekker, Inc., 1979. A textbook.

The textbook I edited contains a very detailed description of my particular punch transplanting technique. In addition, it contains sections by four other physicians who use somewhat different approaches for reasons that they explain. Numerous references are listed. You should be able to translate the medical jargon into everyday English by using the synopsis of medical terms included at the end of this book.

Although this chapter has attempted to give you an outline of what might occur at a typical transplanting session, I want to repeat that there may be considerable variation from practitioner to practitioner. Also, no single approach is the "best." Hair transplanting is a procedure that involves many variable factors—and most of these factors are interdependent. Changes in the number of grafts moved per session, for example, may suggest or require changes in the intervals between operations or changes in the transplanting patterns used. Some doctors prefer to use larger grafts, for example, 4.5-millimeter or 5.0-millimeter grafts instead of 4.0-millimeter grafts. Some do no more than forty or fifty grafts per session. Some prefer to begin transplanting in the middle of the scalp and to move forward gradually in subsequent sessions. (The advantage of this latter approach is that it makes the transplanting less obvious, especially when there is some original hair on the top of the scalp that can be combed over the transplanted area. Its disadvantage is that it results in a prolongation of the treatment period. For individual patients, however, this might be a preferable route.) Numerous other variations in technique are used, depending on what is convenient for both the physician and the patient. All approaches have advantages and disadvantages, and these should be discussed fully with your doctor during your first consultation.

You now leave the doctor's office, but not for very long. Your next appointment is scheduled for twenty-four hours later.

7

After the Operation

The First Twenty-Four Hours

Immediately after the operation, the numbness of your scalp and the sultanlike turban on your head are the only indications that you've undergone hair transplant surgery.

But one or two hours later, when the freezing effects of the anesthesia have worn off, you'll probably feel a mild, aching sensation in the areas operated on. As I mentioned earlier, most patients rate it as no worse than the pain you experience after a dentist has worked on your teeth or gums (see Chapter 9). If you take a few headache pills, the pain disappears, and it is almost always totally gone by the time you wake next morning. For about one patient out of every fifty, the pain may persist for a few days (rarely longer) and requires a prescription painkiller. You may be one of the unlucky few, but the odds are strongly in your favor that you won't be. I want to stress, however, that there's no need for *any* postoperative pain—just ask your doctor for a stronger pain pill.

Twenty-four hours after your operation, you return to the office for bandage removal and cleaning.

The accumulation of dried and clotted blood is carefully washed away with a gauze swab that has been soaked in hydrogen peroxide, a disinfectant. The grafts are checked to make sure they're positioned exactly as they were prior to bandaging. If a plug has popped up a bit, it can be set back into place. If a graft has rotated and is now angled in the wrong direction, it can be removed and put in the proper position. Fortunately, the grafts seldom need to be adjusted if dressing and bandaging have been done properly.

With your bandage removed, you are probably now worrying about how much the operation will show when you go out in public. You can usually be totally reassured as far as the donor site is concerned. Surrounding hair can be combed over to conceal the empty spaces where the hair plugs were removed (Figs. 30A and 30B).

Eventually these spaces fill with scar tissue which contracts over a period of three to twelve months. What begins as a four-millimeter hole will usually end up as a scar one to two millimeters wide. Although hairless, such a scar is not noticed unless one actually looks for it by parting the hair in the donor site. Patients always find it difficult to understand how it's possible to take so much hair from a donor area without leaving the hair looking much thinner than it was originally. The explanation lies in this decrease in scar surface area. As a result there is ordinarily much less bare skin left than you would have expected. The effect is little *apparent* change in hair density (Fig. 26).

Incidentally, you usually have to lose at least 50 percent of the hair in any given area before other people notice that you are "thinning."

As for the recipient site, it's often possible to camouflage it quite soon after transplanting by strategic brushing and combing, provided that the patient has enough hair of his own to maneuver with. A few patients can do this as soon as the bandage comes off. A word of caution: When combing or brushing fringe hair over newly planted grafts, avoid catching the edge of a plug and dislodging it. If this should accidentally happen, call your doctor immediately. The plug can be reinserted if it's intact and relatively uncontaminated. It takes seven to ten days for plugs to become fairly firmly anchored; in three weeks, they're completely secure.

If you have very little hair left in the recipient area and not enough hair to comb over it, the grafts will be easily visible for one to four weeks, depending on how well you heal. Usually the crusting is off by one to two weeks and all that's left is a faint red or pink circle at the site of each graft. There is also an awkward period from about the fifth to the eighth month, when two sessions are growing clumps of hair in an otherwise bald area. This problem is discussed in greater detail a few pages farther on.

Some patients ask about wearing a hairpiece following their operation, especially if they've been accustomed to wearing one. I have two reservations. First, I think that the use of a hairpiece should be avoided for seven days following surgery because the warmth and moisture under it increase the risk of infection. Second, although there are no scientific studies to prove or disprove this, it's my impression that hair growth is not as good if the transplanted sites are immediately covered with a hairpiece. Years ago I let my patients wear hairpieces within twenty-four hours of surgery, so I feel that I'm in a fair position to judge. Once again, I tend to be conservative and prefer to be overcautious. Many doctors allow their patients to wear hairpieces as soon as the bandages come off (the next day), so if you want to wear one, ask your doctor in advance what his policy is.

Naturally, a hairpiece should not be attached with adhesive tapes on recently planted hair grafts.

Postoperative Swelling

Beginning two or three days after the first operation, nearly all patients experience some degree of swelling on the forehead and sometimes around the eyes. This usually lasts for two to five days. It can be very slight or severe, depending on the individual and on how many grafts were transplanted. When small numbers of grafts are transplanted, for example, fewer than thirty, you are unlikely to have any swelling. However, if you have a large area to transplant, it is rarely worthwhile to do small sessions, as many more treatments are then required. The potential benefits should be weighed against the potential disadvantages. In view of the fact that the swelling is only temporary—usually lasting no more than two to seven days—it's usually wiser to have more plugs done per session and to accept some temporary swelling rather than increase the number of appointments in order to avoid swelling.

In some cases, the swelling can be bad enough to cause blood vessels around the eyes to burst, giving the patient a real black eye, or "shiner." This happens in only about one out of every fifty patients and nearly always only after the first operation. Although it looks bad, the condition is quite harmless and clears up by itself. Many doctors, including myself, advise patients to arrange for a holiday or a week off work after the first transplant if at all possible—just in case they're the unlucky ones to get black eyes.

For some unexplained reason, there is nearly always less swelling after subsequent sessions. It's not uncommon for a patient who experiences a great deal of swelling after the first operation to experience no swelling or virtually none after all the rest. The only exception to this general tendency occurs if a period of a year or two elapses between hair transplants. In that case, patients tend to experience swelling of equal severity on each occasion. One way to reduce swelling is by applying ice packs. Another is to remain vertical as much as possible for a few days following the operation. That means sleeping in a reclining chair or propped up in bed on three or four pillows.

Some doctors administer hydrocortisone-type drugs in order to reduce swelling. Although, in my opinion, none of these drugs have been conclusively proven to be effective, a sizable number of fine physicians strongly believe in them.

Swelling is no problem whatsoever when the area being transplanted is the crown of the head. This is because any swelling that develops goes down the back of your neck, where it isn't noticed, rather than across the front of your forehead and face, where it's clearly visible.

Physical Activity

You should give up active sports for at least a week after your hair transplant. Strenuous exercise causes perspiration, and the moisture and warmth provide a fertile breeding ground for infection. Again, in the course of violent exertion—such as playing tennis, volleyball, or squash—you might accidentally dislodge grafts that are still struggling to take firm root in your scalp. Vigorous sports can also produce a significant rise in blood pressure that can cause freshly transplanted hair plugs to pop up.

Patients are usually advised not to exercise for seven days and to avoid shampooing for three days. I also suggest no sex for the first few days, but I sometimes have my doubts as to whether this rule is followed.

The Future Schedule

It usually takes four operations to solidly fill any given bald area (Fig. 39). If you're like most patients, after you've completed one transplant session you still have three to go. At each of the four sessions, from 80 to 120 or more plugs can be transplanted—whatever number are necessary to fill in your bald spot.

Most physicians leave an interval of at least six weeks between the first and second transplant sessions. Although subsequent operations can also be spaced six weeks apart, some of us prefer to wait three or four months after the second session before proceeding to the third. This delay makes it possible to see how the hair is distributed over the surface of the grafts transplanted in the first two sessions. The hair within grafts sometimes grows in more to one side or another of the grafts, instead of being evenly distributed across the surface. If the space between two grafts is filled before their hair has grown in, the new graft used would be just large enough to reach the edges of the previously placed grafts and could not take into account possible empty portions in them. The result is a small gap between clumps of hair—and, for example, an all too common, unnatural, toothbrushlike effect in the hairline. On the other hand, waiting until hair grows in the first grafts (three to four months) permits the distribution of the hair within those grafts to be seen, so that if the hair does not reach the graft edges, slightly larger grafts can be put in to overlap the empty portion of the

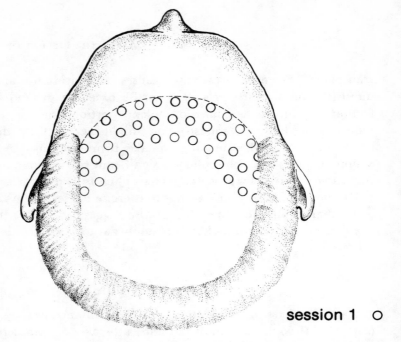

session 1 ○

Fig. 39. Typical approach to solid filling of an area. Timing: second session, six weeks after first session; third session, six to sixteen weeks after second session; fourth session, six to sixteen weeks after third session. Note: some physicians following this general pattern use intervals of as little as three weeks (advantages of a slower approach are covered in the text).

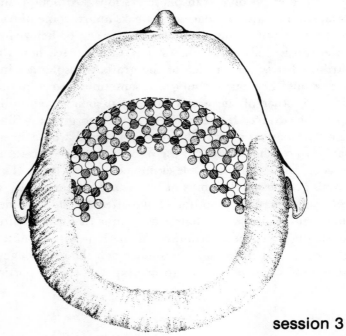

session 3 ◉

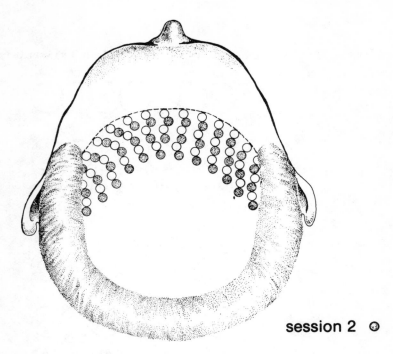

session 2 ◉

While a three row per session pattern is shown here, four or even five rows can be used in most patients if a U-shaped pattern is employed.

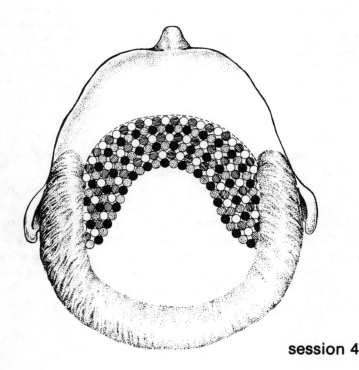

session 4 ●

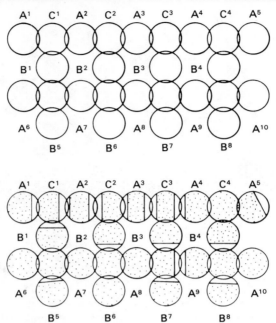

Fig. 40A. The dots represent new hair growth. The third session (C) was done before any hair growth occurred in the first two sessions (A and B). When hair growth did occur, gaps could be seen between clumps of hair, for example, between C3 and A4, despite an allowance that had been made for this possibility by a slight overlapping of grafts. This individual's hairline will look something like a toothbrush.

previous plugs (Figs. 40A and 40B, and Figs. 41A–41C). For the same reason, it's wise to allow another four months to elapse between the third and fourth sessions.

Aside from frustrating the patient's desire to get as much done as quickly as possible, the main disadvantage of the slow approach outlined above is that it makes for a cosmetically awkward period from the fifth to the eighth month after the transplanting is begun. During this time, the hair transplanted in the first two sessions has grown in fairly well, but hair transplanted in the third session has not yet begun to sprout. The coarser, darker, and denser the hair is, the less pleasing the appearance. This temporary unsightliness can

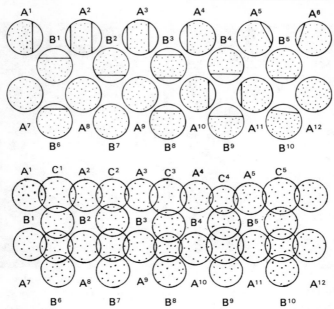

Fig. 40B. Here the operator waited until hair in the first two sessions had grown in before continuing with the third session. Thus the hairless portions of the A and B grafts were clearly evident, and larger grafts could be used in the C session (for example, between A1 and A2, A3 and A4, A5 and A6, and so on). When hair growth extended to the edge of the A and B grafts, because of an allowance for slight overlapping, smaller grafts could be used, e.g., between A4 and A5, A9 and A10, and so on. Use of the same-sized grafts in these sites would have removed some of the hair previously transplanted. The jumble of graft sizes also minimizes any tendency to an overly regular and, therefore, unnatural-looking hairline.

be partially or wholly masked by patients with a reasonable amount of hair left in the recipient area and by patients who have long hair on their rim that can be combed over the grafts. Patients who wear a hairpiece can use it as camouflage. Other patients shave off the newly growing hair until the hair transplanted in the third session is ready to grow in.

As indicated earlier, some patients find these long intervals unacceptable, and all of their sessions are scheduled about six weeks apart. Their hair will still grow well if the other rules of good transplanting are followed. Technically, however, the slower pace is preferable, and it should be followed whenever it is practical to do

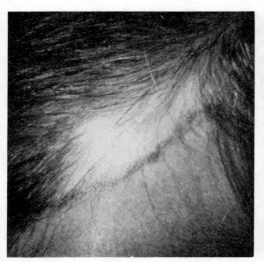

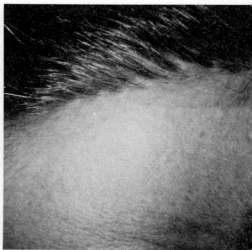

Fig. 41A. New hairline marked in with grease pencil just behind some fine hairs still present.

Fig. 41B. Five and one-half months after transplanting began. Two sessions growing.

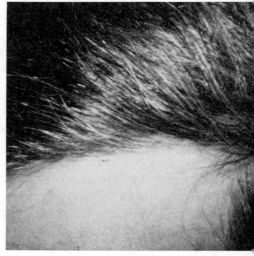

Fig. 41C. Appearance fourteen months after transplanting began, with hair combed up to expose the hairline.

so. In the interests of achieving a better final result, it's probably worthwhile to endure a slight cosmetic problem for a few months.

A variety of patterns and time schedules are used to cover large areas of baldness. Figures 42–46 summarize some of these in schematic form. In practice, the exact patterns depicted in the schematic drawings are rarely used, but you should be able to get the general drift of things from the figures.

Many doctors ask patients to return to the office for a reassessment about six months after the final session. At that time, it may be decided that a further operation is advisable. This is called a "filler" or "blender" session. It is intended to enhance the patient's appearance by filling in or enriching certain areas with strategically placed small grafts. When the slow approach I prefer is used, a filler session is rarely necessary. When a faster approach is attempted, it is almost always required.

How Soon Will the New Hair Grow In?

You can spare yourself a lot of disappointment and frustration by not expecting too much in the way of hair growth too soon after starting.

Once transplanted, the hairs within the plugs may appear to be growing. But in reality they're slowly being thrust out. Within two to eight weeks, nearly all of them will have been shed. After a long pause — eight to sixteen weeks — new hair growth begins. Hair will grow faster in some plugs than in others. Again, individual hairs within the same graft may take anywhere from two to five months to start growing. An average plug contains eight to fourteen hairs, though occasionally a patient with exceptionally good donor sites might have twenty and even more hairs per graft.

The texture of the transplanted hair is usually similar to that of the donor area from which it was taken. Sometimes, however, it initially grows in coarser than the original hair. After a period of six to eighteen months, it regains its natural texture (Figs. 47A–47D in the color insert).

About eight to nine months after your first session, your hair growth will look significantly fuller and richer — an observation that will most likely be confirmed by comments from your family and

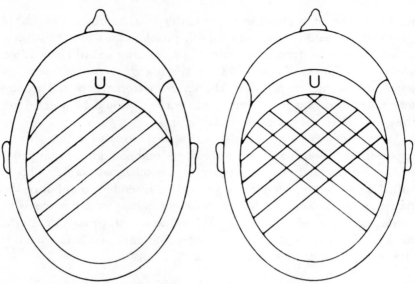

Fig. 42A. Center of the U and left "ledge" transplanted six weeks after any session to U (Figure 39). All of the following sessions behind the U are also to be done approximately six weeks after any session to U.

Fig. 42B. Six weeks after Figure 42A.

friends. From this point forward, your appearance will improve steadily and rapidly. Twelve to fifteen months after your initial operation, you'll be enjoying the full cosmetic and psychological rewards of hair transplantation.

How to Manage Your Hair during and after Transplanting

Hairstyling is important. Not only can it aid you in camouflaging work being done during the course of treatment, but it can also

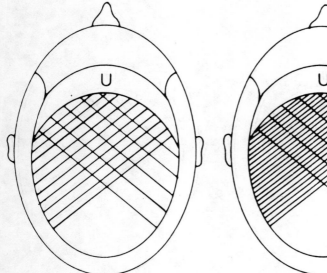

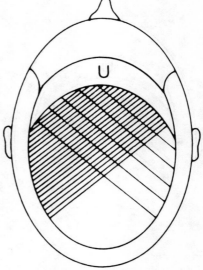

Fig. 42C. Six weeks after Figure 42B.

Fig. 42D. Six weeks after Figure 42C. or . . .

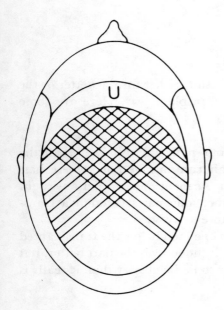

. . . Fig. 42E. Six weeks after Figure 42C.

Each session consists of seventy-five to one-hundred grafts.

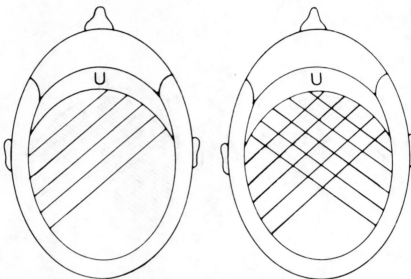

Fig. 43A. Center of the U and left "ledge" transplanted six weeks after any session to U (Figure 39). All of the following sessions behind the U are also to be done approximately six weeks after any session to U.

Fig. 43B. Six weeks after Figure 43A.

affect the appearance of the final result, either for the better or the worse, no matter how good the transplant was. Here are some useful hairstyling techniques:

Lower Part. Try "parting" your hair slightly lower than the area transplanted. Parting the hair can only be done where hair growth is totally even and uniform. As mentioned earlier any slight tufting becomes quite obvious when one parts through a transplanted site, and this should therefore be avoided.

If you part your hair one-half to one inch below the transplanted area and comb this extra hair over it, not only is the part better, but the area being covered can appear to be far denser than it really is (Figs. 27A and 27B).

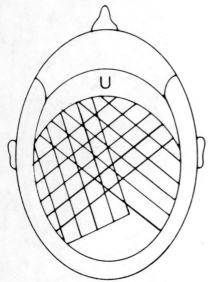

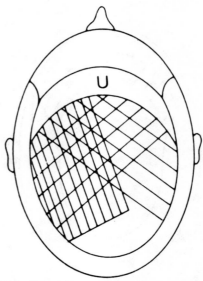

Fig 43C. Six weeks after Figure 43B.

Fig. 43D. Six weeks after Figure 43C or . . .

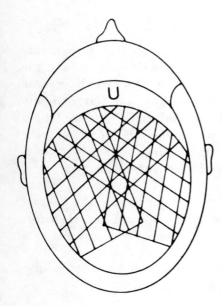

. . . Fig. 43E. Six weeks after Figure 43C.

Each session consists of seventy-five to one-hundred grafts.

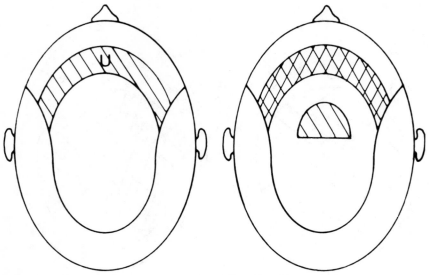

Fig. 44A. First session.   Fig. 44B. Six weeks later.

On a bald person this maneuver may be seen as a desperate attempt to comb a few strands of hair over a shiny head, and the first wind tends to blow the whole thing apart. Once you have some transplanted hair up there, however, you will find that a slightly lower part does not look at all affected and that the transplanted area will be "windproof." A lower part is the most common technique used by patients who have had hair transplanting. It is popular because it is such a simple and effective method.

No Part.   1. Sweep the hair on the temple toward the back of the head and then gradually angle it first upward and then forward, or sweep the hair on the temple upward and forward in a gentle, gradual fashion (Fig. 48B).

2. Wear your hair short and curly. Transplanted hair frequently grows in "kinkier" than the donor area from which it was taken. As

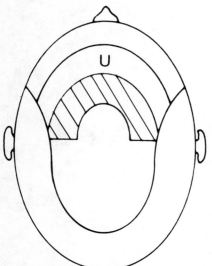

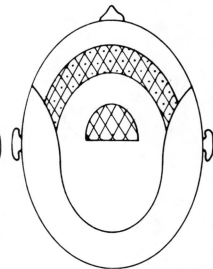

Fig. 44C. Six weeks after Figure 44B, a session has been done in the U-shaped area behind the first U-shaped area.

Fig. 44D. Six weeks or more after Figure 44C. Three sessions have been done in the first U and two sessions have been done in the "island."

Fig. 44E. Six weeks or more after Figure 44D, a fourth session has been done to the hairline on the part side and a second session has been done to the second U.

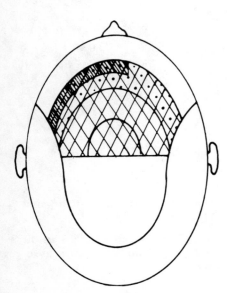

Each session consists of seventy-five to ninety-five grafts.

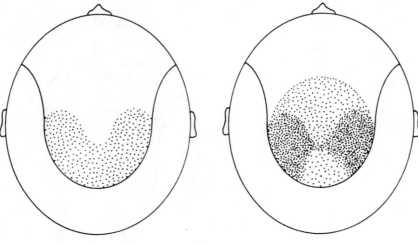

Fig. 45A.

Fig. 45B. Six weeks after Figure 45A.

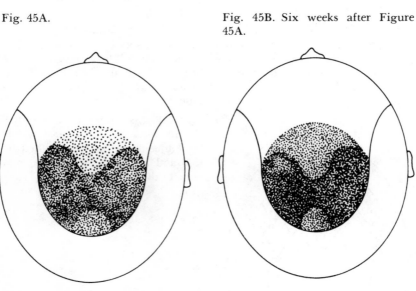

Fig. 45C. Six weeks or more after Figure 45B.

Fig. 45D. Six weeks or more after Figure 45C.

Overlapping Us in the vertex area result in four sessions of grafts to the center, left and right of the vertex, and two sessions to other areas. Additional sessions may be done if necessary.

Each session consists of seventy-five to one-hundred grafts.

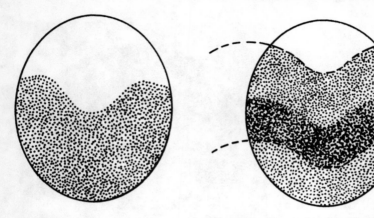

Fig. 46A.   Fig. 46B. Six weeks after Figure 46A.

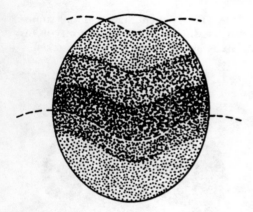

Fig. 46C. Two and one-half to
four months after Figure 46B.

Large areas of alopecia over the vertex can be transplanted by means of this "wave" technique. The fourth session, two and one-half to four months after Figure 46C, is similar to the first, or it can be angled slightly to cover the right side and the rear aspect of the vertex. This results in four sessions to the center vertex, with lighter coverage more peripherally. Additional sessions may be done to thicken any strategic areas.

Each session consists of seventy-five to one-hundred grafts.

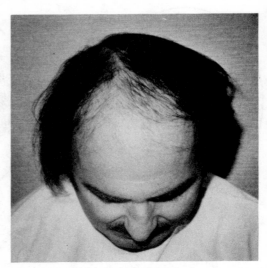

Fig. 48A. This patient had had one transplanting session done on the front of his scalp six weeks before this photo was taken.

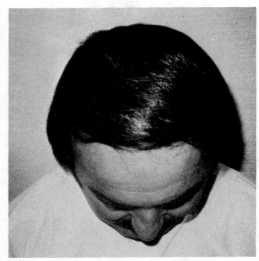

Fig. 48B. By combing his hair forward from his right temple, the patient is able to disguise the operative site. This grooming technique can be used very effectively both immediately after a transplanting operation and in order to make the hair look thicker after transplanting has been completed.

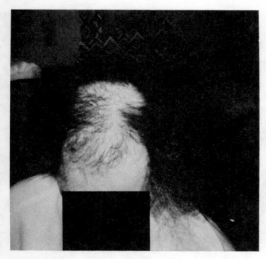

Fig. 49A. A patient before transplanting. Three sessions were used to thicken the front four inches of his hairline. When the patient started transplanting, he had enough hair left to completely camouflage the operations by appropriate grooming.

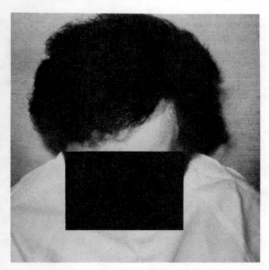

Fig. 49B. The same patient after transplanting. This patient had slightly frizzy hair, so he had a permanent wave done rather than try to fight the hair down constantly.

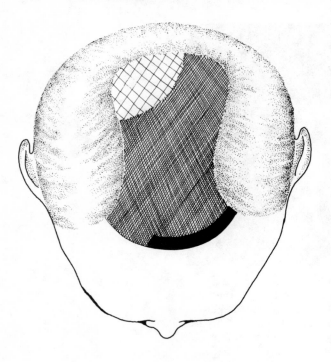

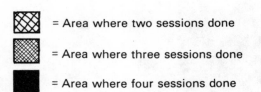

= Area where two sessions done

= Area where three sessions done

= Area where four sessions done

Fig. 49C. Eight sessions, with a total of 582 grafts.

was noted earlier, over a period of six to eighteen months it gradually reacquires the texture of the hair in the donor site, but initially it contrasts with any remaining fine hair in the recipient site. (This is one of the drawbacks of thickening frontal recessions that haven't gone completely bald yet.) Patients who have naturally curly or kinky hair experience an exaggeration of this problem and often

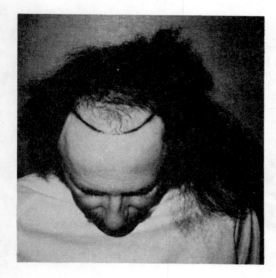

Fig. 50A. Before transplanting.

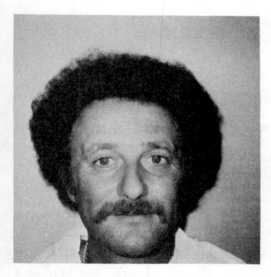

Fig. 50B. The same patient after three transplanting sessions with his hair cut short. After washing his hair he frizzes it up with his fingers, using a messing action until dry. Subsequently a fourth session was done to further thicken the front.

have a considerable amount of difficulty in combing their hair down and keeping it in place after the transplant begins growing in.

The problem, however, can become a great advantage if you will "swim with the current" rather than fight it: that is, don't use a

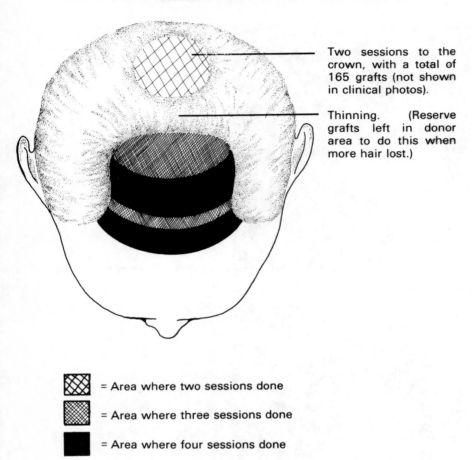

Two sessions to the crown, with a total of 165 grafts (not shown in clinical photos).

Thinning.　(Reserve grafts left in donor area to do this when more hair lost.)

☒ = Area where two sessions done

▨ = Area where three sessions done

■ = Area where four sessions done

Fig. 50C. Four sessions, with a total of 368 grafts.

part; cut the transplanted hair relatively short; frizz it up after each washing simply by running your fingers through your hair in a messing action; or you can even have some permanent waving or curling carried out by a hairstylist. This hairstyle will make your hair look thicker. It is also easy to take care of and will allow you to hide any imperfections in your hairline effortlessly (Figs. 49B and

50B). More and more patients, regardless of hair type, are using permanent waving after transplanting. It's perfectly safe to "perm" transplanted hair. (It's also OK to bleach or dye it if you like.)

3. The "Caesar style," in which the hair is combed directly forward, is very useful in disguising otherwise unsatisfactory hairlines. In addition, combing forward thick hair farther back on your scalp can be very effective in covering any thinning areas between your "crown" and the transplanted front of your head (Figs. 51A-51C).

Regular Shampooing.   Shampooing often enough to minimize the oiliness of scalp hair is a very simple way of increasing the apparent "fullness" of hair. It can also be used to great advantage by patients who are going bald. If necessary, your hair can be washed every day with a mild shampoo. Ionil shampoo, Daragen shampoo, and Redken products are my own favorite commercial brands.

Colored Hair Sprays.   Colored hair sprays are available to color the scalp (not the hair) in areas where hair growth is sparse (Figs. 52A and 52B). The hair is parted to the side in regular rows, and with the spray can about twelve inches away, the coloring is applied in light, brief linear movements. Reflection of light from the scalp is thereby reduced, and the hairs that are present do not stand out starkly against a pale, shiny background.

Your transplant will look much thicker if you use this technique in any area where hair growth is not dense. The sprays are water soluble and come in a variety of colors to match the hair of the individual. Streaks 'n Tips and Top Coverage are the commercial brands recommended in our office.

Blow-Drying.   Blow-drying your hair after shampooing is another simple way of producing more body in your hairstyle. Dry hair generates more static electricity when it is combed, resulting in a better dispersion of hair strands and a fuller look. Incidentally, cream rinses and conditioners oppose this static electric charge and therefore have some negative (as well as positive) effects on hair

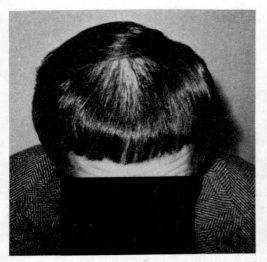

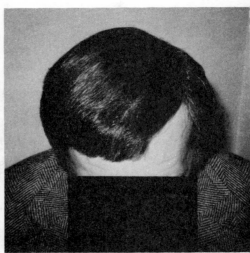

Fig. 51A. This previously bald patient had three sessions to the front of his scalp and two sessions farther back. The sessions are shown growing here. The patient was scheduled to have another session to the front of his scalp and one or two more sessions to the center in order to complete the procedure.

Fig. 51B. Combining his hair in a "Caesar style" allowed the patient to cover the center of his scalp and to thicken the front, to a point where he was entirely satisfied with his appearance. He therefore decided to postpone further transplanting.

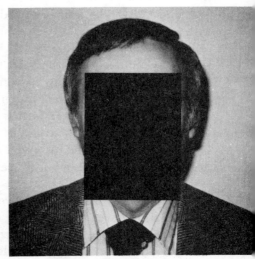

Fig. 51C. Front view of the same patient.

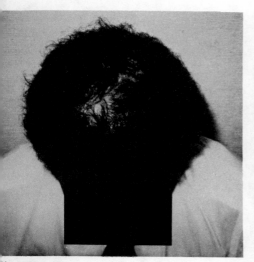 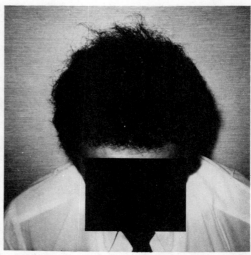

Fig. 52A. Front of scalp transplanted but thinning centrally.

Fig. 52B. Applying colored hair spray to the skin in the thinning area reduced the glare and made the hair appear thicker.

body. I usually advise patients *not* to use hair conditioners unless their hair is in generally poor condition. You should also be careful to choose a dryer whose airflow is not too hot, and to hold the dryer at least six inches from your scalp. Hot or close dryers can dry out and damage hair shafts badly.

Hair Sprays. Although most hairstylists and dermatologists dislike "fixing" hair sprays, such sprays can be used to great advantage once the hair has been carefully washed, dried and combed to maximum effect. As long as you don't overdo it, you can avoid hair damage and the glued-in-place appearance that most people find unattractive. A light spray in strategic areas is all that should be necessary.

8

Complications: What and How Common Are They?

Infection

For the first two to ten days the plugs may look slightly swollen. They may be pale, skin-colored, pink, or even purplish. There should, however, be no pussy discharge or "pus pimples" present.

As has been noted, the incidence of postoperative infection in the recipient area is very small—a fraction of 1 percent. In our office postoperative infection has not occurred at all for the last six years, since we started using antibiotics before, during, and after the operation as a preventive treatment.

Occasionally, after several weeks or months, a small pus pimple may develop adjacent to or on the surface of a graft. This is usually *not* an infection, but represents a site where a small hair spicule was inadvertently left on the plug and is now being pushed out by the skin. Contact your doctor, however, whenever you suspect infection.

The symptoms of true infection are redness, tenderness (it hurts when you touch it) and pain (it hurts without being touched).

If you have these symptoms, antibiotics will be prescribed and the infection should be brought under control very rapidly. You can prevent large areas of infection from developing by simply notifying your doctor at the first sign of any trouble. If infection is arrested early, it should have very little effect on the ultimate growth of hair. If you wait too long to get treatment, however, infection can destroy the hairs in the area involved.

Postoperative Bleeding

Postoperative bleeding in the first twenty-four hours is rare if the patient avoids strenuous exercise. For example, it occurs after one or two operations out of about 600 done each year in our office — and then usually in patients who have bled more than average during the operation and are therefore "suspect." Bleeding after the initial twenty-four hours is even less common. When it does occur, it can be stopped by pressing the bleeding site firmly with a clean piece of gauze or a handkerchief for ten or fifteen minutes. If that doesn't work, the bleeding site can be sutured.

Postoperative bleeding should never be serious enough to be anywhere near life threatening. It represents an inconvenience rather than a mortal danger.

Pain

This "complication" has been covered elsewhere in the book. There are, however, a very small number of people who experience varying degrees of discomfort over a longer time than usual. In fact, sometimes the discomfort can last several months. The pain is almost always limited to the donor area, and it tends to occur in intermittent, short, sharp twinges lasting one to several seconds.

In order to keep the subject of pain in perspective, I would like to remind you that a majority of patients require no painkillers at all after the operation, and that among those who do experience pain, it has usually vanished after twelve to twenty-four hours.

Numbness

Cutting some nerves in the course of transplant surgery causes patients to experience some degree of temporary numbness in the donor and recipient areas. However, it's usually not very bothersome and normal feeling almost always returns in three to eighteen months. Some patients have reported a permanent decrease in sensitivity at one or both sites but these represent unusual exceptions to the general rule.

Itching

Occasional itching in the donor or recipient area can become a problem. A combination of an antibiotic and a "cortisone" cream can be used in such cases. Your doctor will prescribe one for you if necessary. If itching occurs it usually lasts a few days, and it rarely persists for more than two to four weeks.

Graft Elevation

If transplanting has been carried out properly, grafts usually heal flat with the surface of the scalp. Occasionally, however, they may heal slightly higher than the surrounding skin. This is sometimes referred to as "cobblestoning."

Often, slightly elevated grafts will flatten out on their own in six to twelve months. Those that fail to do so, however, can be flattened out by an electric needle, by "dermabrasion," or, occasionally, by shaving their tops off with a sharp scalpel. The important thing to remember is that the final result of transplanting can, and should, be a smooth surface.

Differences in Skin Color

The initial red or purplish color of the grafts gradually becomes a pale pink, and then, over a period of two to six months, it should become the same color as the skin in the donor area.

Unfortunately, the skin in that area has been shielded by its hair from the aging effects of the sun and the environment, and it is nearly always paler than the color of the skin on your forehead. This difference in color may draw attention to your new hairline. Gradually, the grafts will "age" and blend more naturally into the color of the forehead. In the interval, colored makeup or "tanning" agents can be used by the fastidious patient. Tattooing has been used by some.

The easiest route of all is to let the hair in the hairline fall slightly forward—it will want to do that anyway—so that the difference in color is not visible. I also ask patients to pull their hair back to expose the hairline whenever they're sunbathing. They can use sunscreening agents to protect the face and forehead but allow the skin of the hairline to sunburn slightly, thereby speeding up the aging process.

Keloids (thick scars)

Virtually all patients heal properly. However, there is a very small group of individuals who heal in a peculiar fashion, forming large and unsightly scars wherever they are cut.

This problem is most common on the head, neck, and upper chest and arms, and in blacks. If you have a history of healing in an unusual way after being cut, you should bring this to the attention of the transplant surgeon whom you consult. He may advise you against having a transplant. Or he may conduct a trial by transplanting a single plug to see how well or how poorly you heal.

"Arteriovenous Fistulas"

This is the name given to small, blood-filled sacs that form as the result of a vein healing onto an artery instead of onto another vein or instead of shriveling up.

This rare complication nearly always occurs in the donor area. It can be removed surgically, but it will eventually disappear on its own, twelve to eighteen months after the operation.

Poor Results

There are two main reasons that a patient may be disappointed with the results of his transplant surgery. He may find (a) that he's not growing enough hair or (b) that he's growing enough hair but that the cosmetic effect is unpleasing.

Let's deal first with inadequate hair growth. Poor growth of transplanted hair has many causes, and all of them are avoidable. There's simply no reason for your transplant operation to fail if the doctor you've chosen knows what he's doing and if you have followed his instructions carefully.

Let me list the main surgical reasons that transplanted hairs fail to survive: (a) improper cutting of grafts, (b) improper handling and overzealous cleaning of plugs, (c) drying out of plugs due to an inadequate amount of solution in the cleaning dish, (d) sessions that are too large in relation to the pattern used, (e) sessions that are too close in time, and (f) plugs that are too large or too close.

If you're lucky enough to have a relatively loose scalp, you may be able to partially correct a poor hair yield by using alopecia reduction (see Chapter 2) along with additional punch transplanting. A surgeon can remove the least hairy portion and transfer any reasonably growing plugs from this excised section to the remaining areas. This allows you to eliminate a very thin site while thickening a moderately thin one at the same time, but without using up any additional plugs. The grafts which are transferred during this corrective procedure do very well despite the fact that they're being moved for the second time.

The second major kind of disappointment that is experienced by transplant patients relates to their appearance. True, their transplanted hair is flourishing in formerly bald areas, but the overall cosmetic effect may not please them.

Some of these patients feel badly let down because their expectations were unrealistic. You can't expect a transplant surgeon to perform miracles. No doctor on earth can give you back that rich, luxuriant head of hair you had when you were a teenager. If you are attempting to cover a large bald area, there simply won't be enough donor grafts to fill it all in solidly.

These are important matters that should be discussed with your surgeon before the operation—not after. He will give you an accurate estimate of what proportion of your bald area you can fill, considering your supply of donor hairs. If you want to cover a

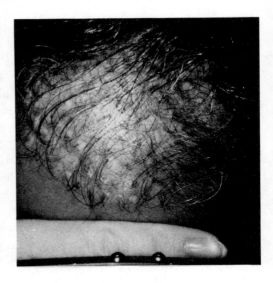

Fig. 53. This patient had 100 plugs grafted at one sitting in a massed pattern that did not adequately take into account circulation to the transplant site. Another 100 plugs were transplanted three days later in the same area. The blood supply to the area was markedly interrupted by relatively large and poorly planned grafts that were too close together. Extremely poor growth resulted.

somewhat larger area, he will also advise you how to make up for a deficit of hair by the strategic placement of grafts (Figs. 23A–23G and 24A–24D) and the use of hairstyling techniques.

In other cases, as has been noted earlier, the fault lies not with the patient but with technical or artistic inadequacies of the doctor. Recently, a growing number of patients have required additional surgery in order to correct poor transplanting results. In fact, that was one of my main reasons for writing this book. Obviously, a lot of people simply didn't know enough about how to find a good transplant doctor and about what was involved in hair transplanting.

Some of these patients were operated on by doctors who believed that the transplanting procedure was simple and that it could be performed without special training and experience. This is far from accurate. Transplanting may look simple, but only the inexperienced believe that it is.

Summarized below are five examples of "transplant failures." In each case, the patient was the victim of an inadequately skilled physician or of a physician who lacked good cosmetic judgment.

Case 1.   This forty-four-year-old patient reported that he had

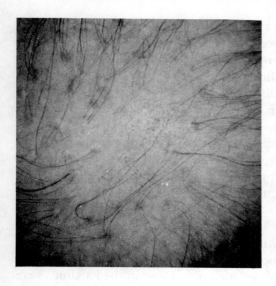

Fig. 54. These grafts demonstrate poor cleaning technique and misdirection, with some adjacent grafts pointing in quite different directions.

very little growth on his bald spot, despite the fact that 200 grafts had been planted in it over a year prior to this photo (Fig. 53).

After questioning him, I learned that the 200 grafts had been implanted into the same general area in two sessions only three days apart. Trying to transplant so many plugs into the same zone in so short a time made failure inevitable. The scalp couldn't suddenly provide a supply of blood sufficient to nourish the transplanted grafts adequately. Hence, hair growth was stunted.

Moreover, the wide spacing used between grafts resulted in an ineffective covering of the patient's bald spot. In order to place grafts close to each other, you have to wait until the first grafts have healed completely and taken root. This patient should have had three or four sessions, spaced at least six weeks apart. The bumpy grafts or "cobblestoning" was also totally avoidable.

Case 2. This forty-five-year-old patient complained about his transplant because it had resulted in only a minor increase in the hair on his bald spot and because the new hair was growing in a strange, unnatural manner (Fig. 54).

He was the victim of at least two errors. I suspect that whoever cleaned the donor plugs before transplanting was overzealous and undertrained. The roots of many of the hairs were probably clipped away along with the excess fat, thereby making sparse growth inevitable. The second mistake was inserting the plugs without paying attention to the direction of hair growth. The result: The hair was growing in all different directions, making it impossible for the patient to comb his meager supply of hair in any reasonable pattern.

Cleaning plugs is a tedious and time-consuming task. It often takes two experienced nurses between sixty and ninety minutes to prepare eighty to ninety plugs. If this part of the procedure is not carried out meticulously, the final result of the transplant can be disastrous.

Case 3.   This young man of twenty-six had two transplanting sessions, both of them done with great care and skill, except for one terrible error: All of the plugs, including those in the hairline, were placed so that the hair grew toward the back of his head (Fig. 55). This created a bizarre appearance, because hair in a normal hairline grows forward. To correct this mistake, it was necessary to remove all the grafts and replace them with properly directed plugs.

Fig. 55. The direction of hair growth in the transplanted area is exactly opposite to that of the patient's original hair. Hair on either side of the recipient site is growing in an entirely different direction from that of the transplanted hair. That hair should have been used as a guide to the correct placement of the transplanted hair.

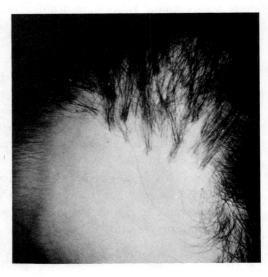

Case 4. This thirty-eight-year-old man was unhappy because his transplant resulted in a hairline that was rather sparse and was situated low on his forehead (Fig. 56).

This unsightly product was the handiwork of a surgeon who was deficient in both skill and aesthetic judgment. Care should be taken to place the first row of grafts in the hairline well back, because, as was mentioned previously, the hair tends to grow forward and it will often appear to be one to two inches lower than it actually is. In the interests of naturalness, patients should be encouraged to accept a somewhat receded appearance. In addition, the grafts were too widely spaced, so that it would be impossible to fill the area in four sessions.

Case 5. This twenty-nine-year-old patient was concerned about his temporal recessions. He asked the physician to eliminate them and to move his temple hair more toward the front at the same time (Figs. 57A and 57B). The most important faults demonstrated here include poor graft direction (in some areas, the exact opposite of natural); elevated grafts, or cobblestoning; poor spacing of grafts; and perhaps worst of all, the attempt to move the patient's temples forward. Transplanted hair grows in far too thickly to produce a

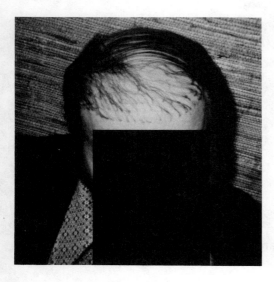

Fig. 56. This patient demonstrates: (a) a hairline that was placed too low (mid-forehead), (b) overwidely spaced plugs, (c) poor hair growth in some grafts, and (d) misdirection of the hair in some grafts.

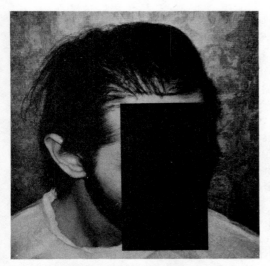

Fig. 57A. This patient's results demonstra
poor graft direction (in some areas it's opp
site to the natural direction); elevated graf
or "cobblestoning"; poor spacing of graf
and perhaps worst of all, an attempt to mo
the temple area forward. It is impossible
produce a natural-looking temple area wi
punch transplanting, and this should nev
be attempted.

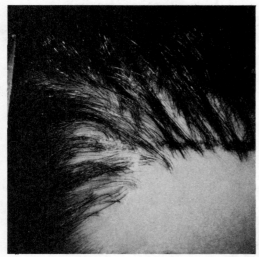

Fig. 57B. Close-up of the same patient.

natural appearance along the front line of the temples. Normally
the hair at this site is very fine and sparse, and there is simply no
way to mimic this with transplanting.

I want to emphasize that these five cases represent a few transplanting failures in a sea of successes. I mention them to underline a bit of advice offered at the beginning of this book: Choose your hair transplant surgeon with the utmost care, because failures in cosmetic operations tend to be highly visible.

Correcting Poor Results

If you've been unfortunate enough to have suffered a poor result because of an unwise choice of physician, don't abandon hope. Start over again by selecting a qualified transplant surgeon, using the guidelines provided in Chapter 3 of this book. You may be surprised by how much he can do for you. After a careful assessment of your hair and your appearance, he may suggest one or more of the following remedial measures:

1. A new hairstyle to make better use of the hair you now have.
2. Additional grafting with your remaining donor hair. You may be pleasantly surprised to learn that you have more left than you think!
3. Alopecia reduction, as outlined earlier, to eliminate sparse areas and thicken others without using up any additional grafts.
4. Moving grafts that are too far forward back to where they should be.
5. Using electrolysis to remove any poorly placed hairs.
6. Flattening bumpy grafts with dermabrasion, an electric needle, or scalpel shaving.
7. Redirecting the hair in some grafts.
8. A flap graft, as described in Chapter 2. This may be used in some cases to correct errors in the mid-scalp or crown.

Don't despair until you've made a last check with someone who knows what he's doing.

9

A Survey:
The Patient's View of
Hair Transplant Surgery
(Patients' Responses to a Questionnaire)

To obtain a patient's view of hair transplant surgery, early in 1978 I mailed a questionnaire to a random sampling of individuals I had operated on during the preceding five years. I received replies from 173 of them. Summarized below are the questions and their answers.

1. *To what extent were you concerned about your hair loss?*
Of course, all of the patients were sufficiently unhappy about their encroaching baldness to seek remedial action. The prevailing attitude among the majority was, "Unfortunately I'm going bald, but fortunately I don't have to put up with it since a medical solution for my problem is available."
About 50 percent of the respondents described themselves as "very" or "mildly" emotionally upset about their hair loss. On the other hand, 50 percent simply preferred not to be bald.
Comments: "I was upset for professional reasons. In the theater business, losing your hair is a serious matter. I felt that a transplant

was an easier, cheaper, better answer to my baldness than the hairpiece I had been wearing."

"I had a thick mop of black hair, and then, within a comparatively short period, it turned grey and I began losing it. This gave the impression of rapid aging, and it bothered me. I thought it would be better to do something positive about my problem, rather than keep worrying about it and become neurotic."

"I was getting very self-conscious about my disappearing hair. Pictures of myself really bothered me. I became so sensitive about my appearance that sometimes I would stay at home instead of going out."

"I do not subscribe to the belief that 'Bald Is Beautiful' à la Kojak. While accepting the inevitability of aging, I feel that the attempt to slow down the visible symptoms is worthwhile."

"I was driving my wife crazy by worrying about what my baldness had done to my general appearance."

2. *Had you previously tried other treatments or remedies for your baldness? If so, what were your reasons for discontinuing them?*

Almost one-third of the patients had previously tried some other method of solving their problem. Listed below is the frequency with which the various methods were tried.

Scalp and hair studios or salons	13%
Hairpieces	8
Hair transplants	3
Hair weaving	2
Hair implants	1
Other	1

The patients described their dissatisfaction with the various kinds of treatments tried in the following terms:

Hairpieces: "Perspired too much" . . . "It made my scalp feel itchy and uncomfortable" . . . "I found the maintenance and upkeep boring and time consuming". . . . "A continuing expense" . . . "Impractical because it would sometimes become loose and even fall off while I was swimming or playing sports or making love" . . . "I disliked its unnatural appearance."

Hair and scalp studios: "I went fifty times, and the treatments were messy and failed to grow hair" . . . "For two years I took treatments with no noticeable improvement to my baldness" . . . "I lost my hair while using the formula they gave me."

Hair transplants: "I had a series of unhappy experiences with another doctor who evidently didn't know much about hair transplanting and knew even less about good doctor-patient relationships. He never seemed to be finished with me."

Hair weaving: "Uncomfortable and unnatural" . . . "It had to be adjusted constantly."

3. *From what source did you first learn about hair transplants?*

Magazines, newspapers, and journals	46%
Radio and TV programs	15
Friends and relatives	15
Physicians	12
Former patients	12

The largest number of patients—more than 60 percent—first learned about hair grafting from the print and broadcast media. By contrast, doctors were the source of information in only 15 percent of the cases. In a previous survey I had conducted, 70 percent of the patients who consulted their family doctor about their balding discovered that they knew more about hair transplanting than the physician. This is sad but understandable. Physicians are primarily involved in general medicine, and unless they have a special interest in the problem of hair replacement, it's unlikely that they would keep abreast of developments in that field. Despite this fact, your family doctor is still the best route to a competent transplant surgeon. He will know where to make inquiries on your behalf and how to assess the competence of the doctors suggested.

4. *To what extent did your family or friends encourage or discourage your having a hair transplant?*

Encouraged me	51%
Discouraged me	27
Opposed	2
No opinion	20

Comments: "Most people I mentioned it to were skeptical."

"My wife said, 'I'll still love you even if you go completely bald.'"

"Some people seemed to regard hair transplanting as a bizarre, secretive procedure in the same league as a sex-change operation. I regard having hair on your head in the same light as having a shine on your shoes at your wedding — it's not essential, but it's certainly preferable."

"My friends felt that it would be painful and expensive and that the results would be unsatisfactory. They said that it was natural to lose your hair and that there was no point in trying to do anything about it."

5. *How would you compare the pain you felt during your transplant surgery to that experienced on a visit to the dentist?*

Less painful	47%
As painful	24
More painful	20
No opinion	9

6. *How many hours of significant discomfort did you suffer following the operation after the freezing wore off?*

0 to 4 hours	42%
5 to 12 hours	29
12 to 24 hours	16
More than 24 hours	12

7. *What type of painkilling drug did you take after your operation?*

No pills	31%
Tylenol-3	38
Headache pills	14

Demerol	1
Not known	16

Comments about pain and discomfort: "The actual procedure was not painful, but the swelling in my head and the stitches at the back of my neck drove me crazy the first few nights."

"Just about as painful as going to the dentist when he works on your teeth and gums. The only difference is that you don't itch for a month."

"Less painful than the dentist—I looked forward to the transplant sessions; I hate going to the dentist."

"One of the most exciting experiences of my life, and it certainly is not at all painful."

"The main discomfort is being bandaged and having to sleep sitting up for a few nights."

"I slept through the whole thing."

8. *Whom did you tell about your hair transplant surgery?*

Absolutely no one	7%
Only my wife	11
Immediate family and close friends	36
Anyone	46

From the above responses, it's evident that patients are not too reticent about discussing their hair transplants. One enthusiastic man observed, "I've told everyone about it. . . . I bother my friends by crowing about it constantly."

9. *How did your family and friends feel about the results of your hair transplant?*

Happy about it	70%
Unhappy	3
Indifferent	18
No comment	9

Comments: "They were amazed that hair can actually grow back in a bald spot."

"Many people are strangely indifferent — maybe they're too embarrassed to say anything."

"Not too many comments from people, but the important thing is that there's been a marked change in me that I'm aware of — I feel better about how I look, and that's pretty important."

10. *How do you feel about the results of your hair transplant?*

Very happy	46%
Satisfied	27
Dissatisfied	4
Not done yet	23

Of the seven patients who described themselves as "dissatisfied," four had not finished treatment for a variety of reasons. It is not surprising that they were dissatisfied with an incomplete transplant. One of these patients continued to lose hair behind the transplanted area and gave up because he felt that he was fighting a losing battle, continually "chasing" a receding hairline.

Some patients are doomed to disappointment because they persist in an exaggerated belief in what hair grafting might do for them and in the rapidity with which they will see results. They simply "tune out" many of the physician's descriptions of drawbacks and limitations during the planning session which precedes surgery. Other patients minimize the cosmetic benefits they've gained from transplants. For example, available donor plugs may be insufficient to fill a large bald spot. This was the case in two of the three completed and "dissatisfied" patients. But it may be entirely possible to improve a patient's appearance considerably by putting hair only on the front of his scalp. In a similar vein, it is not necessary to "chase" a receding hairline indefinitely. Just transplanting the front third or half of a balding top will "frame" your face permanently and make you look ten or fifteen years younger, regardless of any bald spot that is left or is developing farther back (Figs. 10A–10E).

11. *Since your hair transplant, have there been any changes in your*

personality, attitudes, or habits that either you or others have noticed or mentioned?

Feel more self-confident	45%
Feel younger	28
Feel more masculine	3
Drink and smoke either more or less	3
Observed no change	39

Since some patients gave more than one response to this question, the percentage total adds up to more than 100.

Comments: "My close friends have noticed a change. Not concerned with rain, wind, hair spray, wearing hats — all of which were subjects of neurotic concern previously."

"A nice feeling about results" . . . "Feel more free" . . . "More self-confident when meeting people, and this is very important in my career" . . . "I feel younger and have become more self-conscious about maintaining my correct weight — I'm also more clothes-conscious."

"Hasn't basically changed me. I'm the same guy, but I feel happy that I was able to do something constructive about my hair problem."

"The change is within myself. I feel less anxious each time I look in the mirror, which had been very frequent since I began losing my hair."

"I deliver 100 lectures a year, and I know that I no longer present the public with a completely bald head to look at."

"I didn't get it done to effect a personality change. . . . A nice feeling about the results."

12. *Knowing what you do now, would you have a transplant again?*

Yes	91%
Probably	2
Undecided	4
No	3

Two of the "dissatisfied" patients noted earlier felt that they would still probably have a transplant again — despite not being able to fill the whole bald area.

Although the above replies will give you an idea of what patients think about hair transplanting, the replies should not be regarded as being entirely representative of the views of all transplant patients. A survey of this sort attracts more negative than positive replies. On the other side, there is a small group of patients who feel that the procedure has virtually changed their lives, and they answer the questionnaire in too-glowing terms.

The question on painkillers, for example, indicates that 38 percent took Tylenol-3 after the operation. Yet from my experience I would say that the percentage has been closer to 10 to 15 percent, and that, as mentioned earlier, a majority take no painkillers at all.

Perhaps it would therefore be appropriate to conclude this book by sharing with you what I regard as a more representative commentary. It was added to the bottom of the questionnaire by a man in his twenties who was losing his hair prematurely. His words eloquently express the anxiety and the loss of self-esteem that can accompany going bald. But let him speak for himself:

"I think it's very difficult for the nonbalding person to understand the misery of the person who's prematurely losing his hair. He can't help escape the feeling that he's been cheated by Mother Nature. In many cases, he becomes neurotic — the result of helplessly standing by while the size of the bare spot on his head inevitably grows larger and larger.

"I've done a lot of thinking lately about growing bald and hair transplants. Some men accept their fate passively and graciously; others take remedial actions. Julius Caesar and Napoleon both combed their hair in such a way as to conceal their bald spots. Yet, weren't these men brimming over with self-confidence? Would they have gone to a hair transplant surgeon had such a service been available in their time? Did Benjamin Franklin or Benito Mussolini suffer psychologically because they were bald?

"One could go on and on, trying to assess the impact of the balding process on an individual's psyche, self-esteem, and libido. And what are the psychological effects on a person who has had his hair restored to him by transplanting?

"As a person who has been successfully 'transplanted,' I can answer that question. I feel great about it. I was in my twenties and losing my hair. I was very self-conscious of what balding was doing to my appearance — it was making me look much older — and I was unwilling to accept it. I chose to have my hair restored by transplanting, no matter what the cost. If it meant driving an old and inexpensive car instead of a shiny new Buick, so be it, so be it. It's well worth the sacrifice.

"I predict that hair restoration treatments, like transplanting, will steadily become more widely practiced and accepted in the future. And the medical men who are pioneering in this field of therapy will be lauded for their concern.

Glossary

Acetylsalicylic acid—aspirin
Acid mucopoly-saccharide—chemical found in the skin
Alopecia areata—a disease causing patches of hair loss
Anagen loss—loss of hair during growth phase
Analgesia—a state of not feeling pain
Anastomoses—where two veins or arteries join
Androgen—general term referring to any male hormone
Anesthetic solution—"freezing" solution; injected so pain cannot be felt
Anterior—front
Antibiotics—medicine taken to prevent or cure infection
Apnea—stopping breathing
Aponeurosis—fibrous membrane around a muscle
Arterial bleeding—bleeding from an artery
Arteriovenous fistulae—a connection between an artery and vein creating a small lump which has a pulse.
Atrophic—shrunk
Atropine sulfate—drug used to help prevent fainting
Autograft—a graft taken from your own body
Bacitracin—antibiotic ointment to fight infection
Bacteriostatic drug—drug to fight infection caused by bacteria
Betadine—an antiseptic cleaning solution containing iodine

Biopsy—piece of tissue cut out for microscopic examination

Bleeding diathesis—tendency to bleed excessively

Bleeding screen—blood tests done if a problem is suspected with blood clotting

Bleeding time—time it takes for a pin prick to stop bleeding

Bonnie Blue—a solution to mark patterns on the skin

Castration—removal of testes

Catgut reaction—inflammation after use of catgut stitches

Cellular—refers to cells of the body

Cicatricial alopecia—bald area as a result of scarring

Cobblestoning—plugs that have not healed flush with the skin and therefore have left the scalp lumpy

Convulsions—a violent involuntary muscle spasm, e.g., epileptic attack

Cutaneous disorders—a disease affecting the skin

Dermicel tape—a special medical tape that sticks to the skin but still allows the skin to breathe

Diazepam—generic name for Valium (a popular tranquillizer)

Dihydrotestosterone (DHT)—the most powerful male hormone at the cellular level

Donor site—area where pieces of hair-bearing skin are taken from

Edema—swelling

Electrocoagulation—hardening or destruction of tissues by the passages of electrical current through them

Endothelial—cells forming the lining of blood vessels

Epidermis—topmost layer of skin

Epinephrine—an ingredient of the "freezing" solution to make the area stay "frozen" longer

Epithelial—tissue that forms the outer layer of the skin

Erythromycin—an antibiotic which covers a broad range of infections

Erythroviolaceous—pink or purple color

Fibroblasts—cells which produce fibrous material

Fibrosis—an abnormal increase in the amount of fibrous tissue

Field block—method of "freezing" so a minimum of injections are felt

5-alpha reductase—an enzyme necessary for the body to convert testosterone to Dihydrotestosterone

Follicles—the sheath within which hair grows

Forceps—metal instrument to pick up plugs or grafts with

Frontal alopecia—hair loss at the front of the head

Frontal branch of the temporal artery—blood supply that nourishes the front part of the scalp

Full thickness—all skin layers including fat layer

Galea aponeurotica—fibrous covering over skull bone

Gelfoam powder—powder used on a bleeding area to promote blood clotting

Gentian violet—a solution to make a mark on the skin

Genetic—inherited

Granuloma formation—a tumor or lump formed from skin cells as a result of irritation or infection

Hair matrices—roots of hair

Hemogram—blood test

Hemostasis—stopping of bleeding

Hematoma—blood cyst

Hibitane, Hibiclens—an antibacterial skin cleanser

Homograft—tissue taken and grafted onto an individual of the same species

Humoral antibodies—blood cells or substances in the blood that attack germs and foreign material

Hypersensitive—more sensitive than what is normal

Hypertension—elevated blood pressure

Hypertrophic scarring—healing in an abnormal manner with an uneven surface and excessive bulk

Hypertrophy—enlargement

Hypoxia—lack of oxygen

Inferior—lower portion

Intradermal jet injector—an instrument that shoots fluid into the skin without use of a needle

Intralesional triamcinolone acetonide—injection of cortisone-like substance into the skin

Intravenously—injection into the vein

Lateral—sides

Local anesthesia—"freezing" solution placed in an area so pain cannot be felt

Lymphadenopathy—swelling of the lymph nodes

Lymphocytes—cells in the blood important in fighting infections

Male pattern baldness—natural hair loss

Melanocytes—cells which produce pigment

Meperidine Hydrochloride—Demerol (a strong painkiller)

Mepivacaine Hydrochloride (Carbocaine)—a local anesthetic ("freezing" solution)

Metabolic—the basic functions of the body

Metal trephines—metal punches

Methoxyflurane inhalant anesthesia (Penthrane)—drug which is breathed to cause relaxation and reduce sensation of pain

Micropore paper—a type of tape that air can get through

Neosporin—an antibiotic ointment

Occipital branch (of external carotid artery)—blood supply to the back of the head

Parietal and frontal branches (of the superficial temporal artery)—blood supply to the front, sides, and central scalp

Partial thromboplastin time—blood-clotting test

Penrose drain—a rubber tube to drain undesirable fluid build-up from a surgical site

Peripheral blood smear—microscopic examination of a thin smear of blood on a slide

Pigment—colored particles

Platelet count—count of a type of cell in blood that is important in blood clotting

Portwine Hemangioma—a birthmark that is a purple color and is due to abnormal blood vessels

Posterior scalp—back of the head

Prilocaine Hydrochloride (Citanest)—a local anesthetic ("freezing" solution)

Progesterone—a female hormone

Prophylactically—to prevent

Prothrombin time—blood test pertaining to the clotting of blood

Proximal end—the nearest end

Pruritus—itching

Punch graft—a circular piece of hair-bearing skin

Pustule—blister or pimple filled with pus

Recipient area—bald area which will receive the hair-bearing skin

Reepithelialized—regrowth of the outer layers of the skin

Rejection—tissue not accepted by the body and which, therefore, dies

Retroauricular area—area behind the ear

Running sutures—continuous rather than individual suturing of many sites

Scalp hemostats—instrument used to pinch off blood vessels and, therefore, stop bleeding

Scalpel blade—surgical instrument for cutting
Sebaceous glands—fat glands in the skin
Serum hepatitis—type of inflammation of the liver
Session—one hair transplant operation
Skin turgor—rigidity or firmness of skin
Stridor—a high-pitched, noisy way of breathing due to constriction of breathing passages
Subcutaneous—fatty tissue under the skin
Superior—upper portion
Suture—stitch
Syncope—fainting
Systemic toxicity—undesirable side effects (other than allergic) which affect the whole body
Target cells (gonads)—cells most directly affected are in the testes
Target cells (prostate)—cells most directly affected are in the prostate gland
Telogen effluvium—hair lost in natural way but larger than normal amount (in excess of 100 hairs per day)
Telogen loss—loss of hair during resting phase of hair or "natural" loss
Terminal hairs—coarse hair such as is found on a teenager's scalp
Testosterone—the most important male hormone
Tetracycline hydrochloride—an antibiotic
Thrombophlebitis—the formation of a blood clot in a vein
Toxicity—undesired side effect of a drug, other than allergic reaction
Trimming—cutting off unnecessary edges of skin
Tylenol with Codeine—drug to control or reduce pain
Urinalysis—chemical analysis of urine
Vasoconstriction—blood vessels contracting (getting smaller)
Vellus hairs—fine "baby" hair or "fuzz"
Venous or capillary bleeding—bleeding from small veins or capillaries, as opposed to larger veins and arteries
Vertex—crown

Index